I0022766

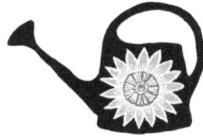

FOOD FOR THOUGHT

Sharing Love, Inspiration, and Connection

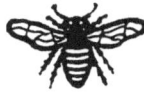

AMY TOBIN

PRAUSPRESS

Copyright 2025 Praus Press

All rights reserved. No part of this book may be reproduced or transmitted in any form or by any means graphic, electronic or mechanical, including photocopying, recording, taping or by any information storage or retrieval system, without the permission in writing from the publisher.

Published by Praus Press

For Sean, Katie,
Olivia and Charlotte

Connecting with you each morning has
been one of the greatest joys of my life.

Sean and Katie, from your very first days, you
have been my whole heart. Olivia, you became
family the moment you walked into our lives.
And sweet Charlotte, you are the newest
light in your Grandmommy's life.
My "word" is joy, and
you embody it.

TABLE OF CONTENTS

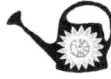

Prologue
–1–

Prologue

Life begins each morning
—Joel Olsteen

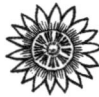

It's been said that the first hour is the
rudder of the day—*Steve Pavlina*

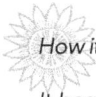

How it began

It began with coffee, though I can't really remember precisely when. As long as we were married, my husband brought me coffee in bed each morning. I loved starting my day peacefully, from the cozy comfort of my bed, a strong cup of coffee in hand. I refer to it as my time to become "one with the world."

When the kids became school age, I added my morning puzzles to the routine. I did the crossword, the jumble, the cryptoquip, all in bed with the coffee my husband brought me.

My entire family indulged me in this routine. I'll never forget being on a sisters' weekend at our family cottage. My sisters brought me printed copies of the crossword since we didn't get a paper there. Early the first morning, I heard a knock at our front door. I went to see who was there only to discover a cup of coffee on the doorstep. My husband has asked my cousin, Mark, to bring it to me since he wasn't there to do so.

I had such a sense of being loved—by my sisters, by my husband and my cousin. I realize now that slow morning rituals laced with love and kindness have always been how I like to start my day.

Over time, work often crept into this sacred space, but I didn't mind. I found I was at my most creative while cuddled up and sipping coffee. In fact, I started referring to work that was done in my "magic jammies" as some of my best.

Then puzzles went digital

When I gave up the newspaper, my puzzles became a digital activity. Starting my day on my laptop is what led me to collecting quotes in earnest, I loved many of the quotes so much that I wanted to see them again and again, to be reminded of their wisdom with regularity. I started calendarizing them.

Now my morning included my coffee, my puzzles and a daily reading of quotes, poems and passages that were meaningful to me.

Over time, they started to stack up. I had quotes that repeated weekly, monthly, annually, I had amassed quite a collection. My quotes were a private ritual that remained incredibly meaningful to me.

As my collection of meaningful quotes, statements, and articles grew, I started to work my quotes into my professional life. I used these quotes as outlines for speaking engagements, as a way to drive home a point with my team at work, and as a framework for my radio show.

Then the quotes moved into my personal life—big time.

After my son graduated from college, he went through a rough patch. He was working in a new job in a city he hated and mending from a breakup. I wanted to comfort him and uplift him without smothering him so I started sending him a morning text with a quote that I thought might help. Soon I added my daughter to the text.

I realized I felt a dedication to putting a good, strong, positive, inspirational and grounding thought in their heads each day. I wanted to keep connected without being overbearing. I wanted to let them know that I loved them so much that they were my first thoughts each day. And I wanted to show them the power of small things done repeatedly.

As the daily texts went on, I gave my morning quotes some context by starting each one with "Mom's Daily Wisdom" and then the quote.

Each morning, I signed off with "I love you both!". As this went on, I abbreviated Mom's Daily Wisdom to "MDW".

Very soon, MDW became "a thing". I loved that I got an "I love you Mom" back each morning. I loved when they would say "Great one Mom" If I was late with it, my kids would call me out on it—"Where's the MDW?"

As I write this, I have sent 2926 MDW to my kids and my daughter in law is part of the text chain, too. I've missed a few days here and there, but that's it, just a few days.

Now it's a calling.

I've known I had to do something with this heartfelt project, and not just because my kids like it. When I would use quotes to frame my speeches, people would approach me afterward letting me know they really needed to hear the particular message that day. I've been so touched by the number of people that will still tell me about one of my quotes or statements that continue to impact their lives.

I have studied the value of rituals, especially the ones that start the day. I know the power of starting with a good, centering thought. It's my hope that this book works for you like it works for me—to start your day with a good thought, a deep thought, or a thought-provoking idea. I hope it's a good thought you can use, and that it's just what you needed today.

Signing off from bed, in my magic jammies, coffee in hand,

—Amy

CHAPTER ONE

Envisioning Your Best Life

*Honing and Owning
Your Life Vision*

Tell me what you eat, and I
will tell you what you are—
Anthelme Brillat-Savarin

I wrote my first life-vision statement over twenty years ago. It was very specific, which is crucial. Every year I take time to burnish and refine it.

I was lucky to have author Keith Ferrazi as a guest on my radio show and I remain inspired by his "personal success wheel". It's a pie chart that includes professional development, spiritual life, charitable endeavors, financial life, physical fitness, etc. Come the first of each year, he reflects and rebalances it.

Inspired, I began to use my google calendar not just to track meetings, birthdays and dental appointments, but to track my life vision and how I really spent my time. It's a check and balance system to make sure I'm living the life I say I want.

Do a personal audit. How do you spend your time? With whom? Doing what? How do you spend your money? Eat? Work? Does it match up with what you want for your life? Tell me what you eat, and I will tell you what you are.

When you see a thing clearly in your mind,
your creative "success mechanism" within
you takes over and does the job much
better than you could do it by conscious
effort or "willpower"—*Maxwell Maltz*

You'll see it when you believe it
—*Wayne Dyer*

Creating a vibrant and detailed mental vision of what you will achieve is as important as the work you do to achieve it.

This isn't "out there" thinking. Numerous studies confirm that athletes who continually visualize their goals have a greater degree of success.

It's not just for sports though. Visualization works in all areas of your life.

Using the power of your mind to "see" your desired outcome moves your emotions, behaviors and even physiological responses in the direction of the vision you've created.

Take a tip from the elite athletes and put this habit into regular, consistent practice.

Sometimes you gotta create what you
want to be a part of—*Geri Weitzman*

Build what you need
—*Brendon Burchard*

The man who follows the crowd
will usually get no further than the
crowd. The man who walks alone
is likely to find himself in places no
one has ever been—*Alan Ashley-Pitt*

I didn't set out to live this way, but this is exactly how I've lived. Throughout my career, I've brought the culture I wanted to work within along with me, negotiated agreements that supported the life I wanted, and, more often than not, successfully built what I needed to thrive.

Brick by brick, conversation by conversation, and intention by intention, you can shape the world you want to be a part of.

I say this often because it's the absolute truth: the cavalry is not coming. No one is going to drop your ideal life at your doorstep. The only person who can create it is you.

And I hope you do—I hope you find yourself in places no one has ever been. Because that's exactly where you belong.

For what it's worth...it's never too late...
to be whoever you want to be. There's no
time limit. Start whenever you want. You
can change or stay the same. There are
no rules to this thing. We can make the
best or the worst of it. I hope you make
the best of it. I hope you see things that
startle you. I hope you feel things you've
never felt before. I hope you meet people
who have a different point of view. I
hope you live a life you're proud of, and
if you're not, I hope you have the courage
to start over again—*F. Scott Fitzgerald*

This is everything. Your life unfolds based on you—your courage, your faith, your perseverance, and your determination to design the life you want. Imagine starting each day with this as your rallying cry.

What happens next depends on what you plan. Set aside time to define what you want in every major area—family, career, health, and relationships. Then, create small, consistent actions to move toward it daily, weekly, and monthly. Check in, adjust, and keep going.

Here's a fundamental truth: without a plan, you can't expect much. Without clarity, you won't see results. So, what do you want out of life? Make it your mantra, your mission, your rallying cry. Then, go make it happen.

The best way to predict the future
is to create it—*Peter Drucker*

Dream of travel? Plan a trip. Save for it. Research it. Pack your bags.

Want to become lean and strong and fit? Pick up a weight and start lifting it.

Want to have a great relationship? Work on it. Every single day.

What you put into life comes back in spades. Create the future you desire, step by step, action by action, thought by thought.

One day at a time.

The things that matter most should
never be at the mercy of the things
that matter least—*Goethe*

When we spend our time, money, attention, and head space on things that are not important to us or don't serve us, it's a slow drain on our soul.

We can't ditch all our responsibilities at once, but we can, moment by moment, keep turning our life in the direction of what matters most.

Navigate your life deliberately and focus on what truly matters to you. Schedule your priorities and let the rest fill in.

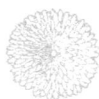

Clarity of vision is the key to achieving
your objectives—*Tom Steyer*

Take stock of what you really want to do with your days, your weeks, your months...your life.

If you take the time to build a foundational vision, stay focused on the things that make you feel most alive, then schedule your time to maximize them, you will have a year unlike any other.

*If you continue to do so, you will have a **life** unlike any other.*

What reason do you have not to create the life of your dreams?

The people who get on in this
world are the people who get up
and look for the circumstances they
want, and, if they can't find them,
make them—*George Bernard Shaw*

When you do things from your soul, you
feel a river moving in you, a joy—*Rumi*

What do you want from your time on earth? Who do you want to spend time with? Be in a committed relationship with? Work for or with? Devote your working life to? What parts of the world do you want to see? What skills do you want to build?

*The first step in activating your plan is recognizing that there will be no knock on your door, no letter in your inbox, no package under the tree that delivers **everything** to you.*

Sure, if you've built a strong network, there will be people who help you, who connect you, and who encourage you. But in this world you need to make things happen for yourself. You're going to have to create it. This may seem impossible, but it's not.

Create a vision of what you want. Review that vision daily. Talk to people who can help. Build the skills needed. Take baby steps each and every day and watch your life start to unfold as you wish it to be.

No one said it would be easy, but everyone knows it's worth it.

Develop a higher vision of your life:
the higher the vision, the greater
the fulfillment—*Deepak Chopra*

You'll never rise any higher than
how you see yourself—*Joel Osteen*

These quotes both reinforce and enhance each other out.

A higher life vision doesn't have to be a grand vision. How you see yourself doesn't have to be exaggerated.

Creating a vision of yourself and your life as something to reach for, work for, strive for is guaranteed to be far more fulfilling than passively accepting whatever happens to come your way.

Regard yourself as capable and worthy. Mean it, believe it, live it. See yourself living the life of your design.

Then go live it.

The key is not to prioritize what's
on your schedule, but to schedule
your priorities—*Stephen Covey*

*Think through your daily agenda and you'll see that some
tasks are essential. The rest should be meaningful to you and
your hopes, goals and dreams. You are the editor of your own
life, so make deliberate choices.*

*At work, are you prioritizing the activities that will move you
along on your desired career trajectory?*

*At home, are you investing time with your community, family
and friends to build the personal life you want?*

Are your self-care routines sacred and non-negotiable?

*Don't over commit. Learn to say no to things that don't align
with your priorities. It's easy to get carried away by a current
of other people's priorities, but the life you dream of requires
that yours come first.*

Find out who you are and do it
on purpose—*Dolly Parton*

I've had many interesting conversations with many people. There's been one common thread: it's a **knowing**.

In some cases, it's been a **knowing** they're in the wrong line of work, relationship or mindset. In other conversations, it's been the sudden crystal-clear knowing they're in precisely the right place, right work, right circumstances. And in others, it's been the bridge between the two.

Knowing it's time. Time to change. Time to go where they have always known they needed to go, but they just had to get uncomfortable enough to compel themselves forward.

One of the best things you can do for yourself is to honor who you really are. And be it on purpose. What lights your fire? What captures your imagination? What makes you come alive? Odds are very good that's the direction you should point yourself. You can come up with a long list of reasons not to do so. You can justify it all day long. That's fine. It just means you haven't hit that point of being uncomfortable enough.

Here's an experiment for you. Ask a close friend, a family member and a colleague to use three words to describe you. Look at the list. Do you recognize the person there? Does it reflect your work and lifestyle? Is it who you are? Are you living your life on purpose?

Each of us has an inner dream that we can unfold if we will just have the courage to admit what it is. And the faith to trust our own admission. The admitting is often very difficult.

What we really want to do is what we are really meant to do. When we do what we are meant to do, money comes to us, doors open for us, we feel useful, and the work we do feels like play to us—*Julia Cameron*

This sounds so simple, doesn't it? Just do what you're meant to do. Easy-peasy.

Of course, it's not that easy, but this particular juice is definitely worth the squeeze.

Pay attention. What lights your fire? What gets your heart racing? What makes you lose track of time? What do people ask you for your help, insight or assistance on? These are all signposts.

*Work is a necessary part of life, and it takes up a good portion of your time on earth. The best way to make that time enjoyable and satisfying is **to do work you love**.*

Yet many people spend their lives doing work they don't even like. Don't be one of them.

Wherever you go, there you are
—*Jon Kabat-Zinn*

It's easy to get caught up in the flawed thinking that if you were in a different relationship, job, town or climate, suddenly your life would be perfect, just as you'd like it to be.

We imagine it's something outside of us that holds the key to—and the responsibility for—our happiness, our success, our wealth. It's harder to think about how we're contributing (or not) to our results. We are the common denominator in our lives.

You can run, you can hide, but wherever you go, there you are.

It begins with your own awakening, your own desire for a life that's not just lived on the surface but is rich and deep and high and wide. For sure, that's how I want to live. So I'm going to keep learning until I take my last breath—*Oprah Winfrey*

Rich and deep and high and wide. I love this vision for life.

You may think it's easy for Oprah to say, but her life certainly didn't start out this way. Maybe she lives this way now precisely because she had this goal. Maybe that awakening led to the rich and deep and high and wide life she enjoys.

I do know that you can bring these qualities to your life in everyday moments. It takes vision, perseverance, and a commitment to banishing the mundane and rejecting mediocrity.

As Vince Lombardi put it, "the man on top of the mountain didn't fall there." It's a climb. Keep climbing 'til you take your last breath.

I learned that there were two ways
I could live my life: following my
dreams or doing something else.
Dreams aren't a matter of chance,
but a matter of choice. When I
dream, I believe I am rehearsing
my future—*David Copperfield*

Even if you can't just snap your fingers and
make a dream come true, you can travel in
the direction of your dream, every single
day and you can shorten the distance
between the two of you—*Douglas Pagels*

Sometimes people say, "I'm livin' the dream" What would that look like for you? Can you define your dreams? It's hard to live them if you don't know what they are. Or worse yet, if you don't have any.

Dreams don't just simply come true. You make them come true. Clarifying them, speaking of them, planning for them, "rehearsing" them, striving to achieve them and traveling in their direction.

Now that's truly livin' the dream.

We've got two lives—
the one we're given and the one
we make—*Mary Chapin Carpenter*

The life you're born into is your starting point, but its potential is finite, limited by circumstance and fate.

Your true potential lies in the life you create for yourself. By definition, your potential goes beyond what you were—or weren't—given. It's in your hands to shape, no matter the hand you were dealt.

Even heirs to great fortunes can't build a meaningful existence from their share of the wealth alone. A purposeful life comes from what you build with intention, resilience, and passion.

It's the life you build on your own which will define you.

Figure out what you're good at
without trying, then try—*Isabel*

Can you easily name your strengths? Do you pay attention to the things people ask you to weigh in on? Can you describe what comes effortlessly to you?

Work to understand what you're truly good at and what you enjoy and be able to communicate it. Are you a creative mind? A pro at problem-solving? A mediator? Maybe you're known for bringing people together or organizing details?

Your talents can take you far, especially if you are keenly aware of them. Working in your comfort zone boosts your chances of success. Working to hone your natural talents can take you even further.

James Clear wrote, "How would my daily schedule change if I did a little more of what I'm great at and a little less of what I'm not great at?"

Don't waste your time on things that don't match your strengths and passions—it's a missed opportunity for both you and the world!

The successful person recognizes his
God-given talents, works relentlessly
to turn his talents into advanced
skills, and uses those advanced skills
to achieve success—*Larry Bird*

Many of the best-known people in the world are famous because somewhere along the way they recognized their God-given talents and ran with it. Bill Gates, Andrea Bocelli, Michael Jordan, Taylor Swift.

We can't all reach superstar levels like this group, but we will come a whole lot closer if we work on developing who and what we authentically are and the skills that come most easily to us.

Diagnose your weaknesses.
Understanding your weaknesses
can end up being the source of
your greatest strength. Those
who understand what's holding
them back are already moving
forward—*Keith Ferrazi*

This is a tough one. No one likes to think about their weaknesses, shortcomings, and flaws.

But we all have them. Identifying them is akin to spotting spinach in your teeth—it can be embarrassing and uncomfortable yet essential for growth.

I've come to understand that it's far better to know and understand our weaknesses and blind spots rather than walking around grinning with spinach in our teeth.

Self-awareness is far more powerful and productive than denial or avoidance.

When you are inspired by some great purpose, some extraordinary project, all your thoughts break their bonds: Your mind transcends limitations, your consciousness expands in every direction, and you find yourself in a new, great, and wonderful world. Dormant forces, faculties and talents become alive, and you discover yourself to be a greater person by far than you ever dreamed yourself to be—*Patanjali*

I find this quote to be tremendously powerful. All the words are full of potential, energy, and the transformative power of inspiration.

Yet, how many of us are spending our time and energy in ways that don't inspire us? How can we pivot back to the things that DO open this extraordinary way of being.

As Patanjali realized, by setting small, achievable goals aligned with your passions, you'll gradually start to make them part of your daily life.

Consistently aligning your activities with your inspirations can and will make you a greater person, by far more than you ever dreamed yourself to be.

Deserve your dream
—*Octavio Paz*

God gives every bird its food,
but He does not throw it
into its nest—*JG Holland*

Listening to someone say they dream of world travel as they watch life from their couch is not nearly as powerful as observing the person who dreams of world travel while scrimping and saving for their dream adventure, researching their destinations, and ultimately booking their next trip.

Dreams aren't entitlements or something that are granted. They're something you chase, something you focus on, something you make happen.

You've got to believe in your dreams and believe in yourself.

But you've also got to get out there and make it real.

Don't ask what the world needs.
Ask what makes you come alive
and go do it. Because what the
world needs is people who have
come alive—*Howard Thurman*

However old or young you may be, you have the entire rest of your life in front of you.

Your calendar is likely still mostly blank. You're in charge of what you do with your available time.

Ask yourself what brings you joy? What lights your fire? Can you be brave enough to create your own authentic life?

Why not book time now for the things you love to do. Make missing them non-negotiable. Let them become your personal rituals.

You deserve it. And the world does, too.

I think that you find your own way. In
the end, it's what feels right to you...
Not what anybody else told you but
the still, small voice—*Meryl Streep*

Learn to trust yourself, your gut, your instincts.

Get quiet and listen to what your "still small voice" (full of immense wisdom) has to say.

You won't steer yourself wrong.

"How are you complicit in creating
the conditions you say you don't
want?"—*Jerry Colonna*

This one's a tough pill to swallow as it forces you to confront some uncomfortable truths.

When you look at the areas of your life that cause you pain or frustration—are you somehow contributing to that?

Take a step back and assess every corner of your adult life: relationships, finances, career, health, spirituality, leisure. Sure, you might not be exactly where you want to be. That's fine. Progress takes time, and effort will bring you closer to your goals.

But what's not fine is sitting back, complaining about the things you can change, and doing nothing about them. Or worse, shifting the responsibility and blame onto others. Ask yourself— how are you complicit in maintaining the very conditions you wish to escape?

CHAPTER TWO

Turning Vision Into Reality

Building Habits For
A Purposeful Life

You'll never change your life until
you change something you do daily.
The secret of your success is found in
your daily routine.—*John C. Maxwell*

Fight this. Or embrace it.

That's the truth, plain and simple.

Don't try to change all your daily routines at once.

Instead, grab one positive habit and commit to it. Once it's baked into your rhythm, add another. Magic awaits.

Improvements are only temporary until they become part of who you are. The goal is not to read a book, the goal is to become a reader. The goal is not to run a marathon, the goal is to become a runner. The goal is not to learn an instrument, the goal is to become a musician. This year, focus on the identity you want to build—*James Clear*

I was lucky to have James Clear as a guest on my show. His book, **Atomic Habits**, is a must read.

The funny/obvious/of-course thing is that we all know what he says is true.

One marathon does not a runner make. It's consistency that we're after. Slow, steady, building each day to the next.

The fastest way to derail any goal is to have too many of them. Don't try to change your whole life at once. If you want to be a reader, read every day, if even for a few minutes.

It takes about ten weeks to form a new habit. Keep going—it will get easier. One day you'll discover it's become your way of life.

Imagine yourself living in a space
that contains only things that
spark joy. Isn't this the lifestyle
you dream of?—*Marie Kondo*

Marie Kondo got us all talking about decluttering, but the benefits of banishing clutter and useless objects is nothing new. William Morris, who died in 1896, said "Have nothing in your house that you do not know to be useful, or believe to be beautiful"

Digging through a junk drawer to find the one item you actually need. Sorting through a closet full of clothes you never wear. Shuffling a messy desk, tanking clear-headed productivity at work. Why do we keep all that stuff? Clutter is soul-sucking.

Well-known organizer Peter Walsh put it so well, "Clutter is not just what's on your floor—it's anything that stands between you and the life you want to be living."

Free yourself from the weight of unneeded (and generally unwanted) possessions. While you're at it, ditch unneeded, unwanted thoughts and habits, too. Don't try to do it all in one day. But do try to do it. Consistently. Isn't that the lifestyle you dream of?

One small win per day is a lot. One of the best pieces of advice from Seneca was actually pretty simple: "Each day," he told Lucilius, you should, "acquire something that will fortify you against poverty, against death, indeed against other misfortunes, as well." One gain per day. That's it—*Ryan Holiday*

One person starts one habit that builds to two habits that builds to three habits that changes an identity that inspires a loved one who influences their peer group and changes their mindset, which spreads like wildfire and disrupts a culture of helplessness, empowering everyone and slowly changing the world. By starting small with yourself and your family, you set off a chain reaction that creates an explosion of change—*BJ Fogg, PhD*

I'm magnetized to the idea and practice of baby steps. Small wins. Every day. We can all do that. And the beauty is, it builds.

If you begin your day with the aim of a win before breakfast, that's a great place to start. What's a small win? That's up to you.

Maybe you meditate for five minutes. Or do a quick yoga flow. Or take your vitamins. Just get that win. And be conscious of it.

Once you get in the groove and turn a morning win into a daily practice, you'll be surprised at how hardwired your brain becomes by looking for and creating more small wins throughout each day.

That feels so good—and feeling good is contagious.

Many of us have made our world
so familiar that we do not see it
anymore. An interesting question to
ask yourself at night is, What did I
really see this day?—*John O'Dononhue*

Making the most of each moment
and ridding ourselves of the toxic
habit of constantly looking forward
to the next thing. Be where your
feet are—*Scott M. O'Neil*

Life is comprised of moments. If you're on autopilot, you'll miss a lot of them. From interactions with loved ones, to the experience of eating good food, or the luxury of waking up in a cozy bed, everything blurs together.

We can't be hyper-aware all the time but finding time to be present—really present—for some portion of every day is a habit worth cultivating. Take a tip or two from Zen monks and:

- *Do one thing at a time. Remember, multi-tasking is no good for you*
- *Do what you do slowly and deliberately—that'll free up your mind to be present and aware*
- *Do what you're doing completely before moving on to another thing: don't leave a trail littered with half-completed projects and tasks*
- *Do less: do what really matters and try to reduce the length of your to-do list*
- *Create space: Leave time and breathing room in your daily schedule*
- *Create rituals: Rituals are focusing and calming. Make your morning coffee or afternoon stretch a sacred ritual where you can center yourself. Make them mini meditations*

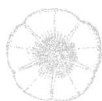

Become who you are
—Friedrich Nietzsche

Imagine being who you truly are. Completely. Utterly, Authentically.

Imagine spending your time, money and attention on what you value.

Imagine comfortably voicing your honest opinions.

Imagine having your authentic thoughts heard.

Imagine surrounding yourself with people who like who you are.

Imagine working for and with people that appreciate the you that you really are.

Now imagine the opposite. Yeah.

Become who you are.

The most difficult thing is the decision
to act, the rest is merely tenacity. The
fears are paper tigers. You can do
anything that you decide to do. You
can act to change and control your
life; and the procedure, the process
is its own reward—*Amelia Earhart*

Making a decision feels so good. Not waffling, wondering, ruminating or second guessing but actually deciding.

It feels even better when we take action on that decision.

Author Mel Robbins wrote a powerful book called "The Five Second Rule" which outlines how mental health struggles and lack of motivation often result in us overthinking our actions.

According to Robbins, it takes just five seconds for the brain to convince us not to do something if it isn't already part of our routine.

We can flip the switch on that by literally counting down 5, 4, 3, 2, 1...then physically taking action before our brains stop us.

Try it out. If you normally hit the snooze button, count down and get out of bed. If you don't want to make that phone call, count down and make the call. Try it in small ways and see how effective it is. 5, 4, 3, 2, 1...GO!

This is the beginning of a new day.

You can waste it or use it for good.

What you do today is important
because you are exchanging
a day of your life for it.

When tomorrow comes,

this day will be gone forever.

In its place is something
you've left behind.

Let it be something good

—*Variation on a poem by
Dr. Heartsill Wilson*

What did you do yesterday? What parts mattered most? What parts mattered least? What parts brought you joy? What did you do for someone else? What impact did you make? What did you leave behind?

As you head out into today, keep those questions humming in your mind. Think about how you'll answer them tomorrow. Let it be something good.

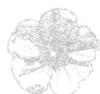

What are the 1–2 things that if
you get them done today, you'll
go to bed content?—*James Clear*

Put that quote on a sticky note and place it on your bathroom mirror.

Decide what those things are, then do them before lunch.

Notice the difference it will make in your day. Keep the sticky note there and keep it going. 1–2 things, each and every day.

It will become a life-changing habit.

First, it is an intention. Then
a behavior. Then a habit.
Then a practice. Then second
nature. Then it is simply who
you are—*Brendon Burchard*

I love what Brendon Burchard teaches.

*This observation is so insightful: for it's how we become who
we become.*

This works regardless of what you "feed" it.

*Make sure that your intention, behaviors, habits and practices are
what you want them to be before they become second nature.*

Course-correct as needed.

Make sure they're making you who you actually want to be.

It is only possible to live happily ever after
on a daily basis—*Margaret Bonanno*

After all, tomorrow is another day
—*Scarlett O'Hara*

If you embrace the idea that each individual day is a mini-lifetime, then treat each day as such and make the most of it. One day at a time.

Get up early so that your morning can begin peacefully. A rushed and frantic morning is a tortuous way to start the day.

Move your body to make it strong and limber. After all, it's the only place you have to live.

Eat good food—not only nutritious foods, but delicious foods. Don't settle for less.

Get quiet—a few moments in meditation makes everything you do smoother all day long.

Do the important things, the things you really must do, first. It'll do wonders for your mindset.

Do fewer things better. Shorten your to-do list and make sure what remains on it matters.

Spend some time each day doing something you love to do.

When you're with people, be with them. Put down your phone.

Do something nice for somebody. There's science behind the fact that you'll feel great about it.

Make your bed a haven and get enough sleep. Count your blessings as you drift off to sleep.

When you complain, you make
yourself a victim. Leave the situation,
change the situation, or accept it.
All else is madness—*Eckhart Tolle*

We've all been hosts to our own pity party, where we bitch and moan about a person or situation.

While this might make us feel better momentarily, it does nothing to improve our situation. Plus it's tiresome for others to listen to.

Snap out of it. If you are truly unhappy in any given situation, do yourself a favor and choose one of Eckhart's strategies. All else is madness.

Nothing succeeds like success.
Get a little success, and then just
get a little more—*Maya Angelou*

So, what if, instead of thinking about
solving your whole life, you just think
about adding additional good things.
One at a time. Just let your pile of
good things grow—*Rainbow Rowell*

You need to be content with small
steps. That's all life is. Small steps
that you take every day so when
you look back down the road it all
adds up and you know you covered
some distance—*Katie Kacvinsky*

Small consistent wins. Little baby steps.

Continuous focus on your own definition of "the prize." Every day.

Just get a little. Then get a little more. Then watch that pile of good things grow! If you keep moving in this way, you will be able to look back and see that you've covered some pretty impressive ground, which would have been hard to do in a single bound.

The moment you accept responsibility
for EVERYTHING in your life
is the moment you can change
ANYTHING in your life—*Hal Elrod*

No one walking this earth is as invested in you as you are. There is no cavalry coming to take responsibility for your life. No one can hand you success—or failure.

No one who can gain experience on your behalf. No one can make you entirely happy. Or make you entirely sad. No one else can clean up your messes.

Your mood? That's on you. Not your spouse, your boss, the guy in front of you in traffic.

Your fitness? Same. Your daily schedule? Ditto.

Circle of friends? You guessed it—that's on you, too.

Taking responsibility means taking ownership of the consequences of your actions and choices. It means doing what you can to learn from and fix things when they go wrong.

*Next time you catch yourself assigning responsibility of your life to another person, give it back to the one and only person it belongs to: **you**.*

The quality of a person's life
is in direct proportion to their
commitment to excellence,
regardless of their chosen field
of endeavor—*Vince Lombardi*

If a man is called a street sweeper,
he should sweep streets even as
Michelangelo painted, or Beethoven
composed music, or Shakespeare
wrote poetry. He should sweep streets
so well that all the hosts of heaven
and Earth will pause to say, 'Here
lived a great street sweeper who did
his job well'—*Martin Luther King, Jr.*

No matter your rung on the great ladder of life, commit to personal excellence.

Learn how to tell a joke, make a toast, offer an apology and take a compliment.

Model the habits and behaviors of people you consider to be excellent. Make your life excellent in all the ways you have available to you and watch the quality of your life expand.

As your level of excellence grows, so will your confidence to create more of it in every area of your life.

Sometimes you get what you want.
Other times, you get a lesson in
patience, timing, alignment, empathy,
compassion, faith, perseverance,
resilience, humility, trust, meaning,
awareness, resistance, purpose,
clarity, grief, beauty, and life. Either
way, you win—*Brianna Wiest*

One of my mantras is "every problem arrives bearing a gift"

I know beyond a shadow of doubt that this is true. I've seen it repeatedly in my own life.

Sometimes we get the chance to learn tough but valuable lessons. Other times we get far better outcomes than we could imagine.

Train your mind to look for the gifts, then realize more often than not, you've won.

Simplicity boils down to two
steps: Identify the essential.
Eliminate the rest—*Leo Babauta*

Focus starts with elimination, improves
with concentration, and compounds
with continuation—*James Clear*

Create scheduled blocks of time where
you do only one thing. Use that block
of time to move your life forward,
to create art, to strategize, to work
diligently on one important activity.
If you don't have blocks of time
already set up in today's calendar to
do things that matter, you're already
losing ground—*Brendon Burchard*

In the big picture of human existence, multitasking is a new thing. How's it working out for us? Not so great.

Humans aren't built for simultaneous thought—we can only hold a little bit of information in our mind at any single moment. So, no matter what we think we're doing, we aren't actually multitasking. We are task-switching, a practice that is stress inducing, wastes time, makes us error-prone and less creative. When we try to juggle multiple tasks, we become overwhelmed with the constant influx of information.

Do yourself a favor, take Brendon's advice and block your schedule to do one thing at a time. Then do it well, do it completely, and take a break before moving on to the next one. Ahhhh. That's better!

Sometimes the smallest step
in the right direction ends up
being the biggest step of your
life. Tip toe if you must, but
take the step—*Naeem Callaway*

I'm fascinated by quotes and adages that seem to be as old as mankind. There are many variations on this theme.

From the Chinese proverb "A journey of a thousand miles begins with a single step" to Desmond Tutu's wonderful "The only way to eat an elephant is one bite at a time." When a message stands the test of time, it's worth paying attention.

Changes that stick, that matter, that move mountains, are generally a series of very small ones that culminate in something bigger than the sum of its parts.

Think about it. Your first workout doesn't make you fit. Your first date doesn't make a relationship. Your first dollar saved doesn't make a fortune.

The best way to achieve all these things is simple: start. And persist.

Each step will get easier and easier until, one day, it's just like breathing.

No person, no place, and no thing
has any power over us, for 'we' are
the only thinkers in our mind.
When we create peace and harmony
and balance in our minds, we will
find it in our lives—*Louise L. Hay*

I'm a believer that your "outer world reflects your inner world"

When our minds are cluttered, chaos spills into our surroundings, and inner turmoil manifests as outer unrest. It's a symbiotic relationship.

When life feels overwhelming, organizing your environment can provide clarity and an opportunity to recalibrate your mindset.

Tap into this practical way to create peace and balance within yourself—and your life.

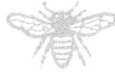

> In every day, there are 1,440
> minutes. That means we have
> 1,440 daily opportunities to make
> a positive impact—*Les Brown*

I love breaking things down into manageable pieces and working backward to tackle big goals.

Say I need to raise $200K for a fundraiser, I look at every part of the event to see how to make each piece collectively contribute to reach the goal.

When I have to pack for a big trip, I'll break each day down to ensure I've got something to wear for all the plans.

If you break a day down into 1,440 opportunities, it's easier to knock something important off your to-do list when you look at the minutes as opportunities for small but meaningful actions. You can return that phone call, do some stretching, step away from the screen, and spend some quality time with your family.

These little minutes add up to days—which add up to our lives. Spend them well.

The difference between good and great is often an extra round of revision. The person who looks things over a second time will appear smarter or more talented but actually is just polishing things a bit more. Take the time to get it right. Revise it one extra time—*James Clear*

Boy, oh boy, can I relate to this one.

In my world it involves getting copy ready for publication, preparing an interview, sending recipes to a client for testing, readying prep trays for cooking segments, creating a run of show for an event.

Overlooking a small detail is less than ideal. The extra round of revision, the second set of eyes, the sign-off sheet, the pre-event meeting—all of these things not only make one appear smarter or more talented, they save a whole lot of grief and regret.

As the carpenter likes to say, "measure twice, cut once".

Catch a wave and you're sitting on
top of the world—*The Beach Boys*

If you think adventure is dangerous,
try routine. It's lethal—*Paul Coelho*

In my early 20's, I had an interior design business in Chicago. One of my services involved walking through a client's home and offering tips to enhance what they already had. I often helped them understand the power of movement in a space.

When you scan a room, there should be a wave-like sense of movement created by the varying heights of artwork, door frames, furniture, curtains, etc. If everything is at the same level, it feels flat and uninteresting. Creating movement adds life to a room.

Another suggestion I often made was asymmetry. Not everything should be perfectly balanced. I would illustrate this by mimicking the scales of justice—arms held out evenly, perfectly equal, but without any sense of movement. It's dull, right?

The same is true for life. It's not all perfectly balanced. Nor should it be. But we can anticipate and prepare for the busy times at work, or the crazy moments with family and schedules. Stock the pantry, catch up on laundry, and let friends and family know you're bracing for the waves ahead. Knowing turbulent times are coming and accepting them, we can surf them. It might even be fun.

When the rush is over, take a break then gear up for the next round. Remind yourself that fear is just excitement without breath—so breathe and remember that balance really is a bore.

"No is a complete sentence."
—*Anne Lamott*

"You have to decide what your highest priorities
are and have the courage—pleasantly, smilingly,
unapologetically—to say 'no' to other things. The way
to do that is by having a bigger 'yes' burning inside. The
enemy of the 'best' is often the 'good.'"—*Stephen Covey*

Throughout my career, people have told me that I have the world's best job—and some days, I wholeheartedly agree. But on other days, my career feels like a giant wheelbarrow full of delicious opportunities, and I find myself trying to devour them all at once. I know I'd savor them more if I could just focus on a few at a time. Yet my time often gets fractured by my desire to be helpful, charitable, and—let's face it—nice.

That's when I remember "Yes means less" from an article by Kevin Ashton on the power of saying "no." He writes that time is the raw material of creation and that saying "no" has more creative power than ideas, insights, and talent combined. "No" protects our time. The math of time is simple: we have less than we think and need more than we know. We're often taught that saying "no" is rude, a rejection, a word reserved for drugs and strangers with candy. But in reality "no" is the button that keeps us focused and on track, while "yes" means less—less time for family, work, and passions. So, how do you start saying no?

Michael Lennington, author of "The 12 Week Year" suggests envisioning a future worth the discomfort of change. He says that to be great, to achieve your full potential, and to execute your plans, you have to be willing to sacrifice comfort. The key is to create and maintain a compelling vision of the future—one that you desire even more than short-term ease. That's how you can align your short-term actions with your long-term goals.

How would your future change if you embraced the idea that "No means no, and yes means less"?

Rituals. The things we do each day,
every day, often arrive without intent.

By the time we realize that they're now
habits, these random behaviors have
already become part of how we define
ourselves and the time we spend.

Bringing intent to our rituals gives us
the chance to rewire our attitudes.

But first we need to see it
—*Seth Godin*

"But first we need to see it". That phrase stopped me in my tracks.

We move in subtle and unconscious ways, allowing routines to begin unintentionally. By the time we become aware of them, they've become habits that define our days—all without much conscious thought.

The tendency to miss these patterns comes from the fact that we are on autopilot. Unless we actively step back and reflect on what we're doing and why, we can become trapped in a cycle of unconscious, unintentional behavior.

While every move we make can't be intentional, it's worth taking a hard look and deciding which things have crept in with no real intention and do a little reshaping as needed. But first we need to see it.

Ask yourself of every dilemma, every choice, every relationship, every commitment, or every failure to commit: Does this choice diminish me, or enlarge me?" As for the answer, that's up to you: The things that diminish you, don't do. The things that enlarge you, do—*James Hollis*

How many times have accepted something—an invitation, a meeting, a project—only to regret it.

What's behind the regret? Laziness? Not likely. Lack of interest? Perhaps. Lack of alignment with who and what you really are? Probably.

What if we were more judicious with our choices? What if we paid close attention to how people and situations made us feel? What if we tried to spend most of our time with the people and activities that made us come alive? Is there any reason we can't make that happen?

We may find lots of excuses, but we'd be hard pressed to find lots of reasons.

The payoff for choosing what makes you come alive is immeasurable.

Health is a relationship between you
and your body—*Terri Guillemets*

I am the first to admit that another glass of wine nearly always sounds like a good idea. Similarly, a greasy, salty French fry is the food of the Gods.

I can talk myself out of a workout so fast it would make your head spin.

But the terrible truth is that wine is going to ruin my sleep and that French fry wants to kill me. The workout? It just might save your life.

Be good to yourself as often as possible so that when you're not, it won't be quite so detrimental.

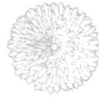

Your heart knows the way. Run
in that direction.—*Rumi*

Self. Help. Helping yourself.

Some folks make fun of self-help. That says a lot about them.

*As the only person who will be with you for your entire life,
helping yourself is smart.*

*Self-help increases health, wealth, happiness, satisfaction, re-
lationships and more.*

Your true self knows what you want and need.

Help yourself and run in that direction.

Trying to improve 1% every day is
better than trying to improve 100%
in one day. If you improve 1% a
day, then in 100 days, guess what?
You're 100% better—*Ken Carter*

I don't believe it's possible to improve by 100% in 100 days, but I do believe it's the general mindset we should adopt.

Instead of trying to become a different person in one fell swoop (a known recipe for failure), what if we tried to just be 1% better than yesterday?

Getting 1% better is a goal anyone can reach. Getting 1% better promises continual growth and improvement. There's no downside to that.

Keep fresh flowers, have a signature look,
have a spot for everything, know what
you like, cherish your style, create rituals
to your liking, romanticize your life, find
magic in the mundane, be an interesting
person, challenge your limiting beliefs,
maximize your existence—*Unknown*

Oh I love everything about this. I want to embody this. It's a lifelong journey.

But I have successfully created rituals to my liking. One of the strongest daily rituals I practice is how I begin my mornings. It's a slow roll into the new day. I like the luxury of an unrushed morning. I'm not the one scheduling 8 a.m. meetings because 10 a.m. is much more civilized.

My morning ritual includes coffee, and lots of it. I bring one black coffee topped with a cappuccino back to bed where I read things that are meaningful to me. I write in my gratitude journal. I do every puzzle available on the New York Times app. I make myself another coffee and review my finances. I shoot a daily text to my kids. I plan my day as I finish my coffee. Then I meditate before hauling myself off to my elliptical or yoga mat.

I really love the mornings, in no small part because I have created and adhere to the rituals that make my mornings delicious. There is magic in the mundane. You can maximize your existence. It's a wonderful, worthwhile thing to do.

Press on. Nothing in the world can
take the place of persistence. Talent
will not; nothing is more common than
unsuccessful men with talent. Genius
will not; the world is full of educated
derelicts. Persistence and determination
alone are omnipotent—*Calvin Coolidge*

It took Thomas Edison 1000 attempts before he perfected the light bulb. JK Rowling's Harry Potter was rejected twelve times before a publisher picked it up. Michael Jordan was cut from his high school basketball team for needing more development.

Imagine if they hadn't persisted?

As Jim Collins said, "Luck favors the persistent." Press on.

Don't promise when you're
happy, don't reply when you're
angry, and don't decide when
you're sad—*Ziad K. Abdelnou*

Strong emotions can cloud your judgment. Being excited can lead to making a major purchase you might regret later. Anger can drive you to end a relationship worth keeping. Fear of failure can lead you down a career path not meant for you.

The key is to acknowledge that emotions are fleeting and not reliable reasons for decision making. They can alter your perspective, make you reactive and lead to regrettable choices. Feel your emotions but put some space and time between them is important.

What's your decision…or is it a response?

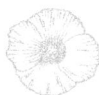

Start putting your heart and soul
into the things you do.—There's a
big difference between empty fatigue
and gratifying exhaustion. Life is
short. Invest daily in meaningful
activities—*Marc and Angel*

We can make just about any activity more meaningful.

I seem to split my time between **mindlessly** completing tasks
and **mindfully** doing so.

Whenever I truly pour my hands and heart into a project, I realize
the difference it makes. From folding laundry to refining an
important presentation, the results when mindfully executed are
just better. When you approach daily life with "the craftsman's
spirit", making things with perfection, precision, concentration,
patience and persistence, you'll see—and feel—the difference.

You're not going to build a billion-
dollar business on a string of bad days.
It has to be a sequence of your very
best days. Your performance is tied
100% to your attitude—*Katia Verresen*

You can replace "billion-dollar business" with a strong marriage, happy family, good health, lush garden, solid reputation. You can replace it with anything that is worth having.

Don't think this means you have to be perfect all the time. It doesn't. But what it does mean is that most of the days you string together must be with the aim of being your very best.

This life strategy has absolutely no downside.

Focus is not a 'business only' thing. Each person has only twenty-four hours per day, and how we spend those hours shows what's important in our lives. The question we must ask ourselves is...Are we focusing on what really matters?—*Mac Anderson*

The master in the art of living makes little distinction between his work and his play, his labor and his leisure, his mind and his body, his information and his recreation, his love and his religion. He hardly knows which is which. He simply pursues his vision of excellence at whatever he does, leaving others to decide whether he is working or playing. To him he's always doing both—*James Michener*

I remember when I realized that weekends shouldn't be so entirely different from weekdays. I was treating my life one way Monday-Friday, and quite another Saturday-Sunday. From what I ate, drank and how I used my time, I was two different people each week.

Think about it: what matters most to you shouldn't be abandoned on the weekend, or during the week! Imagine living in a state of being that is consistently focused on your own personal vision of excellence and bringing that vision to all of your actions and interactions, whether they be work or play.

Every moment of your life is yours and it should look the way you want it every day of the week.

CHAPTER THREE

The Power of Connection

Strengthening Relationships
with Yourself and Others

Learn to have level-headed
conversations with people you
disagree with—*Alan Henry*

Seek first to understand, then to
be understood—*Stephen R. Covey*

It's not easy to be open, kind and good natured when you're speaking with someone with opposing views. In our world right now, developing this capability is crucial. I'm not suggesting it's easy, but I am certain it's worth it.

The key is to not let frustration or anger control you. Don't assume that just because you disagree on one (or many) points that you disagree on everything.

Finding common ground and creating a respectful atmosphere goes a long way in both of you remaining level-headed. Really listening, asking questions and re-stating their viewpoint will draw you into an actual conversation as opposed to a debate. It can also help us to see flaws in our logic, which can make us all more open to compromise. Remember to "attack the problem, not the person" and keep your conversation rooted in facts, and the topic at hand.

Becoming a diplomatic, tactful person who embraces a "win-win" mindset is an honorable way to be. There is no need to conquer every conversation. There's a confidence in being able to allow others their own points of view.

If you're stuck in a negotiation,
figure out the #1 thing that
is truly non-negotiable for
you and then compromise on
everything else—*James Clear*

I suggest you apply this approach to relationships, habits, personal values and boundaries, too.

What are your non-negotiables?

Where do you draw the line? Draw it.

Then compromise on everything else, but not that.

The problem, often not discovered until late
in life, is that when you look for things in
life like love, meaning, motivation, it implies
they are sitting behind a tree or under a rock.
The most successful people in life recognize
that in life they create their own love, they
manufacture their own meaning, they generate
their own motivation. For me, I am driven by
two main philosophies, to know more today
about the world than I knew yesterday. And
lessen the suffering of others. You'd be surprised
how far that gets you—*Neil DeGrasse Tyson*

Everything you need to feel complete begins and ends with you. When you truly get along with yourself—when you're your own biggest supporter and dearest friend—it becomes so much easier to build meaningful relationships with others.

If you're not in the best place with yourself right now, that's okay. Start there. Focus on that first.

Recognize and celebrate your strengths. Be honest about areas for growth and improvement. Take care of your well-being, mentally and physically. Treat yourself like someone you love.

Once you have your relationship with yourself all tucked away, you'll see you already have everything you need to create the life you've dreamed of. That love, that meaning, that motivation?

It's in you.

And the world is waiting.

Never cut what you can untie
—*Joseph Joubert*

In a full life, you'll end many things. How you end them is key.

It is possible to leave a relationship, a job, a friendship or a party without anger, bitterness or destruction. Truly commit to never cutting what you can untie.

We all want to walk through our town, our country, our world, without worrying about who we might bump into. If your conscience is clear and your actions beyond reproach you will gain a sense of peace and freedom not enjoyed by those who burn all bridges. Bridge burners harm their reputations, their relationships, their careers and their mental health.

Throw away your scissors! Become an expert at untying. Rise above.

I no longer listen to what people say,
I just watch what they do. Behavior
never lies—*Winston Churchill*

When people show you who they are,
believe them the first time—*Maya Angelou*

Who you allow into your life,
mind and heart are among the
most important decisions you
will ever make.—*Bryant McGill*

Sometimes your gut will tell you that someone who, on the outside at least, looks like a wonderful person, really isn't. Be wary around them and proceed with caution. Other times you miss all the cues and find out by witnessing an act that shows their true character. How people treat you, treat others, conduct themselves and move through life is indicative of who they really are.

People reveal who they are, loud and clear. And they mean it. We often try to give the benefit of the doubt, or project something better on them, or wish away the negative parts. Don't. People are who they are. You simply cannot change them.

You can however, decide to minimize your interaction with those that don't lift, help, enhance, inspire or improve your life. In fact, you should.

Once we figured out that we could not
change each other, we became free to
celebrate ourselves as we are
—*H. Dean Rutherford (in a letter to his
wife on their 59th wedding anniversary)*

Think about how hard it is to change even one of your own habits. Now imagine trying to alter a core personality trait, or even your beliefs. Next-to-impossible, right?

So why do we expect others to change for us? Why do we assume they should conform to our expectations? That they should bend to our will?

Imagine if Mr. Rutherford and his wife had this understanding from the beginning of their relationship, rather than later in life when hard-earned wisdom most often comes.

Worry about yourself, as they say, and let others do the same.

If someone's behavior doesn't sit well with you, consider taking a step back—whether for a moment or for good, whichever makes the most sense for you.

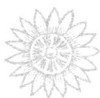

There's only one rule that I know
of, babies—God damn it, you've
got to be kind—*Kurt Vonnegut*

Have you ever witnessed someone do something kind for another person? If you have, you know you get a little boost, too.

Recently, I saw a construction worker helping a woman and her child across a busy intersection. I smiled then, and I smile now, just thinking about it.

Our bodies give us a quick hit of dopamine when we witness, receive, or act with kindness. As humans we love our dopamine.

Go ahead, give yourself a hit through being kind, then enjoy another when you realize your kindness is rippling out to others.

A pause is not a period. It's a comma.
A breath. A moment filled with
so much opportunity to make the
next right decision—*Sally Susman*

Abraham Lincoln wrote what he called "hot letters" He'd release his anger, frustration and emotions into a note, never to be sent. In fact, he'd write 'Never sent. Never signed' on the letter, sparing those he felt anger toward from his wrath.

This practice is a brilliant one. It allows the freedom to say what you really are thinking, to release all your anger, rage, and fury without actually unleashing it on those who don't deserve it. At least not in its most intense form. It lets you cool off, calm down and think better.

To determine what really needs to be expressed and, more importantly, what really doesn't.

To find someone who will love you
for no reason, and to shower that
person with reasons, that is the
ultimate happiness—*Robert Brault*

If you're lucky enough to have someone who loves you unconditionally, you have a gift.

Next to health, loving relationships are probably the most important factor in a happy life.

Knowing the value of love, don't squander it, not even for a minute. Treat it as the precious possession that it is.

Always remember that while finding the right mate is important, being the right mate is equally so. Shower your person with reasons. Every single day,

Be kind, for everyone you meet is
fighting a hard battle—*Ian McClaren*

How often do we interact with others with very little real connection? The cashier is there to check you out. The delivery guy is there to bring your lunch. The customer service person on the other end of the line is there to fix your problem, fast, please.

We rarely consider that everyone we meet is going through some trial. They could be afraid, grieving, sick, worried, anxious, unsure. You don't know what they're going through. We dehumanize each other so readily.

I'm not suggesting you can ease everyone's sorrows. I'm simply suggesting that being human toward another human is always the best choice.

One of the most valuable skills
in life is being able to see another
person's perspective—*James Clear*

You have your way. I have my way.
As for the right way, the correct
way, and the only way, it does
not exist—*Friedrich Nietzsche*

In junior high, I had a teacher, Mrs. Reed, whom I thought was ancient and clueless. I was frustrated by how the kids disrespected her and I just couldn't take it anymore. I marched my 7th grade self to the principal's office and told him all the reasons why she needed to be removed.

To my shock, he called her in and asked me to share my concerns with her directly. Wow. I'll never forget how incredibly hard that was. But I did, she listened, then lifted a coffee cup and asked, "Amy, what side is the handle on?" I replied, "On the right," looking at the principal as if to rest my case.

She calmly said, "I see it on the left. Which one of us is wrong?" Mic drop by Mrs. Reed.

I learned a powerful lesson that day: neither of us was wrong— we just had different perspectives. That insight has stayed with me ever since. Bring a "coffee cup" understanding to all your interactions. (Oh and be grateful to all the best—and worst— teachers in your life, too! All of them have something to offer)

What can you do to promote
world peace? Go home and love
your family—*Mother Teresa*

*Love your family. Love them unconditionally. Love them in every
encounter.*

*Create small rituals and traditions with them. Encourage them.
Inspire them. Forgive them. Make them proud of you. Be proud
of them. Laugh with them. Cry with them. Trust them. Be polite
and kind and thoughtful to them.*

*A strong, positive relationship with your family is one of the
most important elements of a good life. Cherish it.*

We spend precious hours fearing
the inevitable. It would be wise
to use that time adoring our
families, cherishing our friends and
living our lives—*Maya Angelou*

Stop. Stop worrying about the future. Stop dwelling on the past.

Keep your focus on the moment in front of you—this is your life.

Do what matters to you. If everything were suddenly stripped away, the people you'd want by your side would be your family and friends, and the memories you've made together.

These are your true treasures. Love them fully. Don't let what was or what might be cloud what is.

You've got one shot at this life. Make it count. Live it up!

As you know, life is an echo; we get
what we give—*David DeNotaris*

Everything you put out is one
giant boomerang—it comes
back to you—*Elizabeth Rider*

Be the energy you want to attract
—*Terry Pottinger*

When I was in 4th grade, two girls and I formed a little trio which our teacher called the Three Musketeers. For reasons I can't even remember, one of the girls and I decided to start a hate campaign against the third. I'm not proud of this. We passed a note around the class asking other kids to sign it if they hated her. Everyone signed it. Of course, no one really hated her, but it crushed our friend.

The tables turned when she went on her own campaign, and this time I was the target. A note was passed for kids to sign if they hated me. They signed it. Wow. Ouch. It was an awful lesson in "what you put out comes back"

Echoes are everywhere, every day, every moment. The best approach to manage them is to consciously choose what you want coming back at you. Be the person you want to encounter. Raise your energy and you'll see the energy around you rise, too. Lower it and endure the consequences. It's totally up to you.

Set your life on fire, seek those
who fan your flames—*Rumi*

There are people who will never support you
because it's you. Then there are people who
will always support you because it's you.
You just have to find your people—*Unknown*

Choose the people who you allow into your life carefully. Friends, lovers, colleagues—anyone who will occupy a measurable amount of space in your life—with this thought in mind. Those around you can either fuel your passion or extinguish it.

I vividly remember being so excited about what I had learned in a psychology class in college. I was with a group of friends, and I was pumped up. I felt I had found my career path, my calling. One of my friends mocked me, telling me to get my head out of the clouds. While she and I remained friends for many years, there was always a sense she was putting out my fire, smothering me. I finally stepped away from the friendship.

It's crucial to invest in people who ignite your passion, who cheer you on, and who encourage you to keep going. And it goes without saying, be the kind of person to provide them with kindling to fuel their fire, too.

The moment a woman comes home to herself, the moment she knows that she has become a person of influence, an artist of her life, a sculptor of her universe, a person with rights and responsibilities who is respected and recognized, the resurrection of the world begins—*Joan Chittister*

In a real sense all life is interrelated. All persons are caught in an inescapable network of mutuality, tied in a single garment of destiny. Whatever affects one directly affects all indirectly. I can never be what I ought to be until you are what you ought to be, and you can never be what you ought to be until I am what I ought to be. This is the inter-related structure of reality—*Martin Luther King Jr.*

There is a transformative power when a woman embraces her full identity, influence, and potential.

When she truly understands and acknowledges her worth, her ability to shape her life, and her role in the world, she undergoes a profound transformation.

That moment isn't just personal. It has a broader, collective impact. A ripple effect inspiring change in the world around her. When she is who she ought to be, you find that you can be, too. Look around. You'll see it in action every day.

Being aware of a single shortcoming within
yourself is far more useful than being aware
of a thousand in someone else—*Dalai Lama*

Judging a person does not
define who they are. It defines
who you are—*Wayne Dyer*

Don't judge everyone else by your own
limited experience—*Carl Sagan*

*Do you ever catch yourself joining in on the picking apart of someone? It's oh-so-easy to point out flaws in other people. But what's the point? Does it give us some sense of superiority? It certainly doesn't make **us** better or help **us** grow. In fact, it makes us look small.*

What's not so easy is noticing our own shortcomings. Focusing on others' imperfections can distract us from realizing what we need to work on in ourselves.

To become more thoughtful, compassionate, and grounded, we need to leave other people out of it.

Once we learn to shift our energy from judgment to self-reflection, being snarky about others loses its appeal.

Finger-pointing is beneath you. Never,
ever assign blame. Ask instead, what
went wrong here?—*Martha Beck*

This mindset is a game changer. Blaming others might provide a moment of relief, but the aftertaste is nasty.

Flipping the switch to "blame the problem, not the person" will keep your personal integrity intact, while also leading to more permanent solutions—with no bad aftertaste.

It's much more productive to discuss and correct what led to the situation than to throw some poor soul under the bus.

After all, there are likely times in which that poor soul could be you.

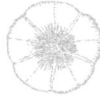

You will learn a lot about yourself
if you stretch in the direction of
goodness, of bigness, of kindness, of
forgiveness, of emotional bravery. Be
a warrior for love—*Cheryl Strayed*

As the Beatles sang, "All you need is love. Love. Love is all you need"

It's all anybody needs—and we need it bad.

What would happen if you approached this day as a warrior for love? If you went just a little bit out of your way to show kindness in every interaction.

Try it. I bet you'll love it. And so will they.

Who you allow into your life,
mind and heart are among the
most important decisions you
will ever make—*Bryant McGill*

Pay attention to your energy level when you are with people.

Who uplifts you? And who drains you?

Who makes you feel powerful, and who makes you feel lesser than?

Time is one of our most precious possessions. Don't give yours to people who decrease its value. Limit relationships that don't nourish, uplift or inspire you.

Think of your life as a sacred space.

Fill it with good people.

Everything that irritates us about
others can lead us to an understanding
of ourselves—*Carl Jung*

There are people in our lives who get under our skin. They rub us the wrong way. They are a pain in the neck.

Once you're done thinking of all the ways they annoy you, look inward and realize that often what we dislike about others exists in us. It's as if we are subconsciously irritated by the reflection of the parts of us that need work, too.

Embracing this allows for a lot more compassion—and a lot less irritation. Give it a whirl.

A loving person lives in a loving world. A hostile person lives in a hostile world. Everyone you meet is your mirror—*Ken Keyes*

Have you experienced a "ricochet"—that moment when your lack of consideration is followed by stubbing your toe or spilling coffee? Or when a kind traffic gesture results in prime parking?

This reminder from the universe that what you put out comes back—often quickly!

Pay attention, and you'll see what you focus on tends to manifest. It's your choice, but life is lovelier when you perceive the world as a loving one.

You are the average of the
five people you spend the
most time with—*Jim Rohn*

It's a worthy goal to have friends that inspire you, lift you, challenge you, support you, teach you—and make you laugh.

Life is too short to spend with those who don't add value to your life.

Want to feel even better in your relationships? Bring those same things to others.

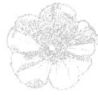

Your task is not to seek for Love,
but merely to seek and find all
the barriers within yourself that
you have built against it—*Rumi*

If you want to be loved, be lovable. That's a variation of a quote from Ovid.

When you're feeling sad, lonely and misunderstood, odds are that you're being a bit unlovable.

What you put out comes back. Ask yourself why. Why are you putting up the barriers?

Self-sabotage is more common than we all admit. Acknowledging our role in feeling unloved is the first step toward attracting love.

To love at all is to be vulnerable. Love anything and your heart will be wrung and possibly broken. If you want to make sure of keeping it intact you must give it to no one, not even an animal. Wrap it carefully round with hobbies and little luxuries; avoid all entanglements. Lock it up safe in the casket or coffin of your selfishness. But in that casket, safe, dark, motionless, airless, it will change. It will not be broken; it will become unbreakable, impenetrable, irredeemable. To love is to be vulnerable—*C. S. Lewis*

Absolutely no one escapes this lifetime without having their heart broken.

It happens to everyone, usually more than once. Remember that giddy excitement of young love? Sure, it ended up breaking your heart, but wasn't that heart-thumping experience worth it?

Grief over the loss of a loved one is shattering but aren't you grateful for the time you did have? Friends, lovers, family members, pets—all bring the chance of heartbreak. It's the price of admission to something really great. Knowing we can't escape it, do it anyway, with all your heart.

I was reminded of what love feels
like and looks like. Love feels safe.
Love feels secure. It feels restful. It
feels like home—*Maria Shriver*

I love this beautiful description of love. It conjures up images of softness, warmth, contentment and light.

This is how I want my family and friends to feel in my home, in my presence, in a relationship with me.

Safe. Cared for. Comfortable. Welcomed. And it's how I want to feel in return.

It's not always easy, but most things this important rarely are.

Always remember that you
are absolutely unique. Just like
everyone else—*Margaret Mead*

While I know myself as a creation of God,
I am also obligated to realize and remember
that everyone else and everything else
are also God's creation—*Maya Angelou*

We live our lives in our own minds and bodies. We see things from our own perspective. We can be generous and kind to others, do our best to understand them, but in the end, we are the center of our own world.

Everybody else is, too. Everybody else wants love, respect, a win, their share, to feel proud.

What if we helped them? Would we also be helping ourselves? This seems like the perfect place to drop the Golden Rule (the answer to just about all of the problems in this world) "Do unto others as you would have them do unto you"

You ARE the other, and the other is YOU.

People pick up on energy. We all carry
energy with us: it's either frantic,
frenetic, and anxious, or solid, calm,
and centered. The energy you bring
to a situation can make a tremendous
difference, be it in your parenting,
in your place of business, or in your
everyday relationships. The tone you
bring to your voice and your words
is critical as well—*Martha Beck*

We've all been there. We've witnessed tensions escalate, almost instantly, after someone brings a negative energy into the mix.

We've also witnessed energy that diffuses and calms vs. invigorates and lifts. It's palpable in all its forms.

Notice what kind of energy you bring with you. Acknowledge that you are 100% responsible for it.

If you're bringing the bad stuff, step back, step out and recalibrate. Then bring your better self right back in.

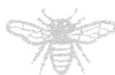

The ability to observe without
evaluating is the highest form of
intelligence—*Jiddu Krishnamurti*

You always own the option of
having no opinion. There is never
any need to get worked up or to
trouble your soul about things you
can't control. These things are not
asking to be judged by you. Leave
them alone—*Marcus Aurelius*

*My recent travel companion was constantly on the lookout. For
what the hotel clerk, the waiter, the cab driver, other drivers
and pretty much anyone we encountered, was doing.*

*It was exhausting to witness. And I didn't like the creeping
realization that I had some of the same tendencies.*

*No amount of looking over another's shoulder, making sure
they're doing things right or second guessing their actions is
going to bring anything good into your life.*

*People are much more capable than we give them credit for. Let
them be. Pay attention to yourself. Ahhhh. That's so much better.*

Remember if you are not speaking
it, you are storing it, and that
gets heavy—*Christina Isabel*

My Mom died when I was in my 20's. As opposed to a sudden unexpected death, there is something about knowing that a loved one is going to die that is both a blessing and a very heavy burden.

I was acutely aware that there would be no second chances to ask and say some of the things I wanted to. I decided not to store it. I spoke it. And it took real courage for me to do so.

I asked my Mom how to cope with losing her, if she would stay connected to me (she did) and her thoughts on life and death. That conversation remains one of the most cherished I've ever had. I like to think it helped her, too.

Most of the things we need to speak are not that intense. But carrying them is heavy nonetheless.

Speak it. Communicate it. Share it.

For me, becoming isn't about arriving
somewhere or achieving a certain aim.
I see it instead as forward motion,
a means of evolving, a way to reach
continuously toward a better self. The
journey doesn't end—*Michelle Obama*

I love how Michelle Obama points out that it's not about arriving somewhere or achieving a certain aim. After all, if that was all life was, that's all life would be.

Instead, it's continuous. Working to become a better version of yourself is ongoing. Learning more about the world and how it works is never ending. Nurturing and tending to your relationships should be a focus as long as you walk the earth.

The same is true about seeking out new experiences and working toward your own happiness and fulfillment. This is no 30-day thing. This is life.

CHAPTER FOUR

A Life of Growth

*Learning, Evolving, and
Becoming More*

The trick to viewing feedback
as a gift is to be more worried
about having blind spots than
hearing about them—*James Clear*

*This. I really learned a lot from this. I talked about it frequently
with my team using the metaphor of letting someone know
they have spinach in their teeth. Or a booger in their nose.*

*Yes, it's hard to say that to another person. Yes, it's embarrassing
to be told it.*

*But what's worse? Delivering the commencement speech with
a hunk of green in your teeth, or knowing you've got someone
who cares enough to let you know about your blind spot. Then
working to correct it.*

*Don't confuse this with taking abuse from people who criticize
and belittle others for kicks. I'm not encouraging acceptance
of that! But finding a person who cares enough to shine the
light onto what you might not see is one of the most valuable
relationships you will ever have.*

*I'll go so far as to encourage you to seek out constructive criti-
cism and feedback. This is great advice from psychologist Adam
Grant:*

"When people hesitate to give honest feedback on an idea, draft, or performance, I ask for a 0–10 score. No one ever says 10. Then I ask how I can get closer to a 10. It motivates them to start coaching me—and motivates me to be coachable. I want to learn how to close the gap."

Sheryl Sandberg also references Adam Grant in this quote about constructive criticism "Taking suggestions from a coach is the whole point of practice. Adam traces his openness to feedback to his past as a Junior Olympic diver. Criticism was the only way to get better."

Of course, it all must be balanced against your own truths and inner knowing. Hillary Rodham Clinton said it so well, "Take constructive criticism seriously, but not personally. Weigh what you hear from others against what you know in your heart to be true."

The very best thing you can do for
the whole world is to make the most
of yourself—*Wallace D. Wattles*

There are so many ways we can make the most of ourselves.

While we can improve our skills and refine our habits, I think any meaningful personal growth begins by being honest with ourselves and facing realities head on.

It comes down to mastering our own minds. It includes not taking other people's actions personally. Assuming good intent and not jumping to conclusions. Trying to understand other people's views before explaining our own. Learning to observe without judging. Being able to harness inner peace and tame outer chaos. Challenging negative thoughts instead of treating them as truths. Letting faith overcome fear. Developing all of these mindsets is the very best thing you can do for yourself— and the whole world.

If a child is poor in math but good
at tennis, most people would hire
a math tutor. I would rather hire
a tennis coach— *Deepak Chopra*

It's true that we all need a base level of competency in many areas and we might need to work on things that don't really interest us but are a necessary part of life. But what's more important is that we should be pushed and encouraged in the areas where we show promise or are gifted.

I love this quote which is often attributed to Albert Einstein (but that may not be true) that really drives the point home: **"Everyone is a genius. But if you judge a fish by its ability to climb a tree, it will live its whole life believing that it is stupid"**

Don't spend your time climbing trees, fishies.

Somewhere, something incredible
is waiting to be known—*Carl Sagan*

The brain is like a muscle.
When it is in use we feel very good.
Understanding is joyous—*Carl Sagan*

Our passion for learning...is our
tool for survival—*Carl Sagan*

We may not all learn (and teach) like the magnificent Dr. Sagan. Imagine if we all set aside 5 minutes a day to learn something new? It could simply be a kitchen hack, a new word or a great short cut, but each time we learn something new we change, literally creating new neural connections. What we learn is ours to keep, no matter what. Learning expands us, improves us, excites us—and makes us much better at cocktail party banter. Something incredible is waiting to be known—by you.

Nothing in life is more exciting and
rewarding than the sudden flash of
insight that leaves you a changed
person—*Arthur Gordon Webster*

Read a lot and be a brilliant
observer—always watching and
searching for new, more efficient,
and faster ways to achieve.
Understand that in order to grow
as a person, you must always
continue to learn—*Peter Economy*

Remember stereograms? They seemed to be random repetitive patterns until you looked at them just right. It would take several tries until a three-dimensional image revealed itself in an uncanny way. Until you saw it, you just couldn't believe it was there. And then? Amazing! There it is!

That's how learning something new feels. Learning releases feel good endorphins and dopamine. Your body literally rewards you for learning. And once you learn something, it's yours to keep and you are forever changed. Here's the thing about life long learners—they are the leaders, the achievers, those living rich full lives. Let's join them.

If you want a radical cure for being a victim, here it is. Victims are dominated by external forces—other people, circumstances—and since outside forces cannot be controlled, it seems natural to give up responsibility for the bad things in your life. "I can't help it" is like a poison seed that keeps multiplying and growing. The solution is to recognize that situations change only after a person quits looking outside and starts taking responsibility.

In effect, you are saying something positive: This is my life. You reclaim ownership of your life once you take responsibility. At the same time, you are stating a simple, inescapable truth. If your life isn't your own, whom else can it belong to? No one else has enough time, money, energy and love to give you everything. Abundance comes from within. When you take responsibility, you accept everything, the good and the bad, as your whole package—*Deepak Chopra*

Personal development starts by taking 100 percent responsibility for everything in your life. This includes the level of your achievements, the results you produce or lack thereof, the quality of your relationships, the state of your health, your income, your debts, your feelings, your thoughts and emotions.—*Meiko Patton*

Some skills don't work when they're average. Responsibility is one of those skills. Average responsibility only holds up when it's easy, obvious, or convenient but quickly shifts the blame when it gets difficult, ambiguous, or inconvenient. True responsibility refuses to shift the blame, especially when the price for responsibility is high. Average responsibility looks for ways avoid responsibility and often invents reasons when it can't find legitimate reasons. True responsibility looks for reasons to take responsibility, refusing to avoid it. Average responsibility isn't responsibility at all.—*Seth Godin*

This is your life. Yours and yours alone. Remove all excuses to the contrary. Give up trying to control anything but your own actions, attitudes and efforts. From the moment you wake until the moment your head hits the pillow, you are in charge.

True, you have authority figures to answer to and obligations to meet, but your attitude toward them is up to you (this seems like a good time to remember that shifting from "have to" to "get to" is a powerful way to think).

True, people and circumstances will trigger your emotions, but your response is up to you. Am I making this sound easy? It's not. Taking 100% responsibility is a load that is tricky and sometimes difficult to carry. It's much easier to tell ourselves that "they did it" or "I couldn't help it". But you know the truth. Own it. Bask in it. Enjoy the freedom responsibility brings.

I've never seen any life transformation
that didn't begin with the person in
question finally getting tired of their
own bullshit—*Elizabeth Gilbert*

I can't help but meet this quote with another: "Wherever you go, there you are"

Nobody else can change you. You know what needs to change. You can deflect it, deny it, avoid it and try not to be responsible for it.

When you've had enough, really truly enough, it's amazing what a large capacity for change each of us has. When you're ready, call bullshit on yourself.

You need to aim beyond what you
are capable of. You need to develop
a complete disregard for where your
abilities end. Make your vision
of where you want to be a reality.
Nothing is impossible—*Paul Arden*

*What's something you want to do that seems impossible?
What would need to change to make it possible?*

*The months and years ahead offers so many opportunities to
amaze yourself.*

*We are all capable of more than we think. It's our limiting
beliefs that hold us back.*

*Taking a deep dive into what we really want for ourselves is
loaded with emotional dynamite. Dream too big and we run
the risk of letting ourselves down. Don't dream at all and we
let ourselves down by default. This year, commit to one area of
your life and create a vision for yourself that feels beyond your
reach. Then keep reaching.*

*In the pursuit of your dreams, even partial progress is a triumph
that will leave you truly amazed.*

You will be the same person in five years as you are today except for the people you meet and the books you read—*Charlie "Tremendous" Jones*

I'm glad I'm not the same person I was five years ago, and I hope I'm not the same person five years from now!

When I think of pivotal moments in my own life and personal development, I can attest that they have been spurred by books or people, or both. All it takes is one conversation or one passage in a book to radically change your point of view and bring forth an idea that could change you forever.

Think Thoughts, Read Books: It's Important To Be Interesting For a worthwhile dialogue we must have something to say. This can only be the fruit of an interior richness nourished by reading, personal reflection, prayer and openness to the world around us. Otherwise, conversations become boring and trivial. When neither of the spouses works at this, and has little real contact with other people, family life becomes stifling and dialogue impoverished—*Pope Francis*

Taking good care of yourself means the people in your life receive the best of you rather than what is left of you—*Lucille Zimmerman*

As a spouse, a partner, a parent, or a friend, being a well-rounded person who takes care of themselves, and their world is part of the bargain.

Take care of your body, mind and spirit. While you're at it, take care of your finances, home and wardrobe. Encourage your spouse, partner, child or friend to do the same.

Give each other your best, not what's left.

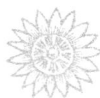

You will never change what
you tolerate—*Joel Osteen*

I used to meet with a small group of women business owners on a monthly basis. (This is a practice I highly recommend. Whatever your area of interest, find (or create!) a like-minded group to talk about it with).

At one of our meetings, my friend Cecilia asked us what we tolerated. This simple question—and a thorough discussion of it—transformed each of us that day. Changes were made to businesses, habits and even a marriage. Wow.

What do you tolerate? Why do you do so? What can you do about it? How would it change things if you no longer tolerated it?

If you can talk about this with someone in a real, true conversation, you might just act on making the changes needed. I hope you will.

Hearing "no" doesn't mean "never."
The only things you can do are to
constantly pursue growth...and
make sure you're prepared to walk
in the room—*Antoinette Robertson*

We all hear a lot of "no's" in our lives. That's what makes the yesses so special!

Let the no's skim past you. Don't get hung up in them.

The magic in this quote lies in making sure you're prepared to walk in the room. What do you need to learn from the no's to walk in that room and get a yes?

I suggest that you entertain
considering the possibility that
you are a powerful and creative,
compassionate, and loving spirit.
Now that may seem a lot, but try that
on for size. And if you find that it
doesn't fit, if you find that there is a
distance between who you are, you
think you are, and what you say and
what you do and the way that you
behave, and a powerful, and creative,
compassionate, and loving spirit,
then also consider that distance is the
distance that you have to travel. That
is your spiritual path—*Gary Zukav*

*The distance between who you are and "who you are being" is
where all the growth and awareness happens. Shrinking that
distance is a lifelong pursuit.*

You cannot solve a problem on
the same level of awareness that
created it—*Albert Einstein*

It's hard to get beyond conventional thinking when you're faced with a problem. But often, to solve it, you really do need to step out of the usual mindset and perspective that led to the problem in the first place. New solutions require a different way of thinking and an expanded awareness.

One of the best ways to get there is to get other people to think with you. Brainstorming sessions, where ideas can be shared without judgment or restriction, are so helpful. The more perspectives you can bring to the session, the better. Gather people from different backgrounds, ages and careers to talk through your problem. You'll see it in a whole new way. In my career, I've loved participating in brainstorming sessions, especially those in fields completely unrelated to mine. I've seen the amazing problem-solving power of a diverse group of minds coming together.

Work to build your own tribe of mentors and advisors. . Watch how they help you to improve the way you approach obstacles in both your personal and professional life. You'll see that great minds don't actually think alike. And that's a powerful thing.

Never underestimate the power of belief when it comes to fulfilling your dreams. I can say with no hesitation that every person I've ever met who has achieved any degree of success has one thing in common: they believed with all their heart they could do it—*Mac Anderson*

I have never encountered a more powerful phenomenon in my life than that of the self-fulfilling prophecy. You become what you believe you will become. And what you believe you will become is influenced mightily by the expectations of others—*John Pepper*

If you expect the battle to be insurmountable, you've met the enemy. It's you—*Khang Kijarro Nguyen*

Your beliefs shape your entire existence.

Ask yourself if you are living expansively, or if you are limiting yourself.

How can you reshape your perspectives to see limitless possibilities instead of restrictions? How can you build the self-confidence to grow without overestimating your abilities?

Tell yourself, tell your family, tell your friends: you can do it.

You can. You will.

Every positive change—every jump to a higher level of energy and awareness—involves a rite of passage. Each time to ascend to a higher rung on the ladder of personal evolution, we must go through a period of discomfort, of initiation. I have never found an exception—*Dan Millman*

There's always a cycle like the cycle of seasons. There's a death and rebirth cycle where you let go of your old identity. Anytime a major change happens in your life, your identity has to let go of the old model. Then you go through a period of feeling very chaotic. Then your dreams start to come in, both night dreams and daydreams. You start to imagine a different future. Then you enact the different future that feels good. Then you perfect it. Then, sure as you're born, another wave of change will come in, and you'll do it all again. Each time you go around, you go forward; like in a screw or a vortex pattern. There's that rhythm. There's a rhythm of change. When I stopped fighting that, my whole life became doable for the first time—*Martha Beck*

Recognizing and accepting the trickier elements of life makes everything easier.

Growth isn't always a joy ride. Change isn't always smooth. Both are worth the discomfort, especially if you are fully clear that the discomfort is part of the process and to be expected.

No one starts as an expert. Initiation is real.

If you can begin to anticipate it as a sign of things to come and step into the flow of it, your whole life just might become doable.

Let me never fall into the vulgar mistake
of dreaming that I am persecuted whenever
I am contradicted—*Ralph Waldo Emerson*

For most of us, this is a tough thing to welcome. Believe it or not, sometimes we are wrong. Sometimes people have a different opinion, perspective, approach or solution than we do. And sometimes they'll let us know.

It doesn't have to mean anything more than what it is. A different way.

It certainly doesn't have to mean it's an attack on your character, intelligence or general value as a human being. Cultivate the acceptance that this is true.

Remind yourself of one of Don Miguel Ruiz' Four Agreements: "Do not take anything personally." It'll save you a world of hurt and angst.

Don Miguel Ruiz' Four Agreements

- *Be impeccable with your word*

- *Do not take anything personally*

- *Do not make assumptions*

- *Always do your best*

Odds are, you've never been to prison...but as humans, we're masters at creating our own. Our prison may be the shame of our past, a desire for perfection or our need for acceptance. The walls might be the potential we haven't realized, a loved one we hurt or even a conversation we never got a chance to have—*Seth Godin*

Elephant handlers train baby elephants by placing a chain around their leg, then attaching it to a stake hammered into the ground. This simple but effective set-up keeps them from wandering away.

When they're full grown, this flimsy arrangement still keeps the elephants in place even though they could easily snap it. What could hold back a baby elephant can't hold back a grown one, but the conditioning is there and the adult elephants don't challenge it. This is the ultimate limiting belief.

Break free from your flimsy stakes and chains. Challenge your prison walls. They're both of your own making and neither is stronger than you.

Divide each difficulty into as many parts as is
feasible and necessary to resolve it—*René Descartes*

Think of almost any problem like a family meal.

If I need to feed my family, first I have to decide what I'm going to feed them.

Do I have the skills needed or do I need to research how to create the recipe? Do I need to practice? Do I need help?

Do I have all the tools and equipment needed?

How much time do I need to get the items ready by my deadline (dinner)?

Then I need to make a list of all the ingredients, making sure not to miss anything.

What food do I have on hand? What food do I have to get?

How will I get to the store to buy them?

If I encounter the need to make substitutions, do I have a plan in mind?

How much will it cost? Does the cost fit my budget?

I need to transport the items back to my home, where I need to wash them, chop them, measure them and prepare them according to the outcome I want.

All these steps result in solving the problem of what's for dinner. To solve successfully you really can't skip any of them.

Most any problem can be approached the same way. What's the solution and how do you get there, step by step? Break it down and it becomes much easier to solve.

You must clear out what you don't
want, to make room for what you
do want to arrive—*Bryant McGill*

Making space. Clearing a path. Making room. Each involves clearing mental, physical, and emotional clutter. This is not woo-woo thinking; clutter and excess in any area of your life can be distracting and obstructive.

Adopt a consistent practice to clear your mind, whether through meditation, walking in nature or practicing qigong.

When you return to the demands of daily life, approach your thoughts as if you're selecting from a menu. Choose only what serves you in the moment and set aside the rest—they will still be available later. You just don't need them now—and certainly not all at once.

Use the same approach for your feelings. Focus on what is helpful now.

For physical clutter, once it's removed, managing mental and emotional clutter becomes much easier. Breathe freely and let what you do want arrive, with plenty of space to do so. Then take good care of it.

Imagine how you want to feel at the
end of the day. Start working towards
that now—*Lin-Manuel Miranda*

*The worst way to spend an evening is ruminating over all the
things you didn't complete, didn't give it your all to, or simply
didn't do.*

*When you tick off all the ways you didn't live the life you
envision for yourself, maybe you missed your workout, had a
petty, unresolved argument with a loved one, went through
the drive-thru for lunch, didn't prepare well, or left a stack of
pressing matters on your desk to greet you tomorrow.*

*Roll back the tape. If you want to have a relaxed evening and
peaceful dreams, set yourself up for success. Plan your day
carefully. Don't bite off more than you can chew.*

*Give yourself moments to renew and refresh throughout the
day. Periodically ask yourself, "Is what I'm doing right now in
line with how I want to live/feel/be?"*

*If your answer is no, ask yourself, "Then why the hell am I doing
it?" Constantly course-correct to get to where you want to feel
at the end of the day.*

The ending is everything. Plan all
the way to it, taking into account all
the possible consequences, obstacles,
and twists of fortune that might
reverse your hard work and give the
glory to others. By planning to the
end you will not be overwhelmed
by circumstances and you will know
when to stop. Gently guide fortune
and help determine the future by
thinking far ahead—*Robert Greene*

The time you want the map...is before you
enter the woods—*Brendon Burchard*

*Planning and preparation are key components to a successful
life. Things run more smoothly, you'll experience less stress
and actually save time by identifying potential challenges and
solutions before they happen.*

*If you don't set your intentions, determine your goals and
define your ambitions, life will do it for you.*

Get clear, get your map and get going.

You can change in an instant. You
can change your mind. You can
change your timing. You can change
your approach. You can change
your words—*Karen Maezen Miller*

Have you ever realized you've painted yourself into a corner?

*It might be in an argument with a loved one. Or halfway through
a book you just don't enjoy. Or any number of situations where
we resign ourselves to seeing through something we don't
mean, don't like, don't want, isn't working.*

*You can walk away. You can end it. You can start again. You
can revisit. You really can change in an instant.*

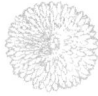

The time to worry is three months
before a flight. Decide then
whether or not the goal is worth
the risks involved. If it is, stop
worrying. To worry is to add
another hazard—*Amelia Earhart*

*If you are making a plan, making a move, taking a risk, or in
any way stepping out of your norm, the best thing you can do
is make a solid plan, then explore its potential pitfalls.*

*Once you've done both, if you still want to move forward,
worrying is every bit the hazard Amelia alludes to. It doesn't
just not help, it harms. Worry saps your mental and physical
health. It erodes your confidence, leads to negative thinking
and makes it harder to focus and think clearly.*

*Put the energy up front and once you've decided the risk is
worth the reward, go for it without worry or fear.*

Marriage is hard. Divorce is
hard. Choose your hard.

Obesity is hard. Being fit is
hard. Choose your hard.

Being in debt is hard. Being
financially disciplined is
hard. Choose your hard.

Communication is hard.
Not communicating is hard.
Choose your hard.

Life will never be easy. It
will always be hard.

But we can choose our
hard. Pick wisely

But we can choose our hard.
Pick wisely— *Devon Brough*

Easy choices, hard life. Hard choices,
easy life—*Jerzy Gregorek*

Every choice carries its own weight.

*Work toward the positive and the hard will become easier over
time, making everything else lighter, simpler.*

*The alternative? Negative choices lead to heavier burdens,
complications, and dead ends. Choose your hard. The amount
of work is the same.*

Fire can burn your house down
or it can cook you dinner each
night and keep your house warm
in the winter. Your mind is the
same way—*Brianna Wiest*

When he was a young athlete, my son often got carried away in the intense emotion of sports.

I used to tell him that he was like lightning. Without focus, he could be destructive. But if he could "chain" his lightning, he had everything he needed to be a powerful force.

Take that same passion, talent, and drive, then tighten it up to turn it into a powerful laser-like force.

Your thoughts are just like that. If you let them run rampant, they can be destructive. But if you channel them, focus them, train them—wow, now you've got powerful options.

A fact is information minus
emotion. An opinion is information
plus experience. Ignorance is an
opinion lacking information.
And stupidity is an opinion
that ignores a fact—*Unknown*

We receive a lot of information every day.

Some facts, some opinions, some distortions and even some lies. Every day.

Our task is difficult. We need to do our own research, our own analysis and, here's the hard part, i.e., not skew the facts to match our own opinions.

Work on that and you won't find yourself in the sorry state of holding "an opinion that ignores a fact". You're too smart to be that stupid.

You need judgment not
impulse. Brains not balls—
Tommy Baxter in "Your Honor"

When I was watching the show "Your Honor", I was so struck by this line that I paused the show to write it down.

Impulsiveness and impetuousness have been a lifelong challenge for me. It's an odd situation for someone who is also such a strategist and planner.

I've learned (often the hard way) that while acting on impulse can be both good and bad (and sometimes incorrectly perceived as courageous), using measured judgment is the far better way to go.

It takes strength. It takes patience. It requires listening to others, asking questions, and waiting to decide.

Truth be told, learning to use good judgment actually takes way more "balls".

When I feel lost and can't make a decision, I just stop and get quiet. I take a time-out. I ask myself, "How does this feel? What do I want my life to be like?"—*Kim Cattrall*

When everything is moving and shifting, the only way to counteract chaos is stillness. When things feel extraordinary, strive for ordinary. When the surface is wavy, dive deeper for quieter waters—*Kristin Armstrong*

When considering a new project or opportunity, one of the first questions to ask is, "How do I want to spend my days?"

Make as few choices as possible that violate your answer.

Many opportunities seem exciting but actually give you less of the life you want—*James Clear*

The importance of taking a moment to pause when life feels overwhelming or uncertain can't be overstated. Stillness is the antidote to chaos. Intentionality is key in creating the outcome, and the life you want. Rather than rushing into solutions, choices or decisions, pause. That's where the peace and clarity reside.

In my own experience, I've found that pausing is crucial to making any significant decision. The moments of regret I remember are those when I acted under pressure or ignored my own feelings. That's when I'd find myself with less of the life I want.

Now I try to begin negotiations with the practice of explicitly saying "I never make a decision without taking a pause," It helps me lay down the ground rules and expectations for myself and those I'm interacting with that my choices are led by clarity. It's a super small yet powerful statement that can change the way you operate.

Say out loud that you're a person who takes a pause, and then take it.

Much of our suffering is caused by our false perceptions and attachment to mental images. We assume things to be true without really knowing whether they are true or not, then create a world of hurt for ourselves and others—*Joseph P. Kauffman*

When I look back on all these worries, I remember the story of the old man who said on his deathbed that he had had a lot of trouble in his life, most of which had never happened—*Winston Churchill*

Can you recall a time that you assumed a scenario that didn't occur—or your assumptions about what would occur were completely incorrect?

Of course you can. In fact, you can probably recall a whole slew of them. It's an element of human nature worth challenging.

Remind yourself of the scientific and philosophical principle of Occam's razor. The simplest explanation is usually the best one. Your headache is more likely due to dehydration than a brain tumor. The noise you heard was probably a car backfiring, not a bomb. The response you're waiting for is more apt to be because they're busy, not ignoring you.

Remind yourself to think objectively. Don't assume anything—and don't take on baseless worry. Most of it never happens.

Don't find fault.
Find a remedy
—Henry Ford

What if firefighters had to figure out who started the fire before working to put it out?

And then gave them a piece of their mind before starting up their hoses?

Fault finding is not helpful in the moment. Solving the problem is.

Truth is ever to be found in simplicity,
and not in the multiplicity and confusion
of things—*Sir Isaac Newton*

In character, in manner, in style, in
all things, the supreme excellence is
simplicity—*Henry Wadsworth Longfellow*

Simplicity is the ultimate
sophistication—*Leonardo da Vinci*

In the building of a basic
wardrobe, we cannot go wrong
if we strive for simplicity and
perfect fitting—*Elsa Schiaparelli*

Simple can be harder than
complex; you have to work hard
to get your thinking clean to
make it simple—*Steve Jobs*

I love quotes because they distill big ideas into simple, powerful messages. Their clarity cuts through the noise, stripping away the unnecessary.

Simplicity is more than an aesthetic or practical option; it's a mindset.

It's about understanding what matters most, eliminating distractions, and focusing on the essentials. Whether in food, art, technology, or even a wardrobe, simplicity lets the true essence of things—including you—shine through.

Have no single point of failure. Have
no single path to success—*James Clear*

*The quality of your life cannot hinge on one thing. Every
element of your life needs a work around, an alternate path,
another option. Every failure must be met with another go, in
another way.*

*Think about it: successful investment portfolios are diversified,
healthy diets are varied, winning sports teams fill their rosters
with players that bring a variety of strengths.*

*Use this understanding to your advantage. It's really as simple
as "Don't put all your eggs in one basket". Ever. Make having a
backup plan your plan.*

Don't be afraid to fail big, to dream big, but remember dreams without goals are just dreams and they ultimately fuel disappointment. So have dreams, but have goals. Life goals, yearly goals, monthly goals, daily goals. I try to give myself a goal everyday—*Denzel Washington*

The word "goal" can spark anxiety in people. I think it's because we take too large a view and often think only of lifelong goals, bucket list goals, big, huge mammoth goals. And those might be dreams. I really like Denzel's last sentence. "I try to give myself a goal every day".

Achieving a small daily goal, making it a touchstone for the day, can pave the way for a larger goal for the week. Achieving a few weekly goals can give you clarity to define—and achieve—a goal for the month. And, you guessed it, if you can achieve a few monthly goals you will be ready to tackle a goal for the year.

I think the key to turning goals into powerful personal tools is to make them super small and achieve them consistently. As you build the size and scope of your goals, make the increase incremental.

I read about a trainer who has her clients start by laying out their workout clothes the night before. And then NOT working out. The goal is simply the preparation. Easy, right?

Next, they put the gear on each day, but don't work out. Still totally doable.

The next goal is to exercise for 2–3 minutes. Bam! Goal achieved. Each workout added a bit more time and a bit more intensity and ultimately a bit more frequency.

Breaking a goal down into manageable steps is the way to get there.

Take baby steps. Go slow, but go steady.

Set yourself up to actually achieve your goals.

If you think prevention is difficult,
try response—*Unknown*

It's far easier to keep a bucket of water close by where a fire may start than to battle the blaze once it spreads.

Easier to fill your tank now than to trudge miles for fuel later.

Easier to address conflicts before they become unbridgeable, to apologize before it's too late.

Life becomes infinitely smoother when you invest in preparation instead of scrambling in reaction. Prevention isn't just a safeguard; it's the basis for peace and progress.

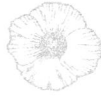

Greatness happens when the person
with the wild imagination collaborates
with the person who knows how
to get things done—*Simon Sinek*

*Whether a friend, a colleague or a family member, this combo is
unstoppable and worth working toward having in your own life.*

Which one are you?

*Find your match and nurture the dynamic because when a duo
like this is in action, people can't help but stand back and clap.*

On the days you only have
40%, and you give 40%, you
gave 100%—*Jim Kwik*

I love this compassionate statement.

Remember to cut yourself some slack.

Not all days are going to be your best days, but doing your best with what you have on any given day is one of the surest ways to have more good days ahead.

Give 100% of whatever you've got, every day.

Being valuable and useful is all you ever need to do to sell things. Help people out. Send interesting posts. Write birthday cards. Record videos sharing your ideas for growing their business. Introduce people who would benefit from knowing each other, then get out of the way, expecting nothing in return. Do this consistently and authentically and people will find ways to give you money. I promise—*Colin Dowling*

Isn't this the Golden Rule rephrased?

How many times and in how many ways has it been said throughout history? Do unto others as you would have them do unto you. Whether in your work or your personal life, stepping into this way of being creates something lovely, for all involved.

The first step to getting out of a hole
is to stop digging—*Trevor Moawad*

When my daughter was a teenager and going through some rough times, I told her to think about problems like being dropped into the middle of a lake. You can splash and sputter and wear yourself out, increasing your likelihood of sinking.

Or you can take a deep breath and swim slowly, steadily to shore and sit on the bank to collect yourself.

When you're in a proverbial hole, swim to shore.

CHAPTER FIVE

The Happiness Blueprint

Cultivating Joy, Gratitude, and a Positive Mindset

What is the most enjoyable
five-minute stretch of your day?
And how could you lengthen it
to ten minutes?—*James Clear*

I had a yoga teacher who asked, "How can you make yourself
10% more comfortable?" As someone who loves to lounge
on the couch to read, nap or watch TV, I followed her advice
and added more comfort with my "lazy table" which slips over
the couch cushion and allows me to reach for my coffee—or
wine—with ease. Cozy throws and pillows amplify the comfort
well beyond 10%!

What small moves can you make to bring more comfort,
pleasure and satisfaction into your life—and your home? How
can you extend the time that means the most to you?

Tending to your personal comfort and enjoyment makes life
much more comfortable indeed.

It's a helluva start, being able
to recognize what makes
you happy—*Lucille Ball*

There can be no happiness if the
things we believe in are different
from the things we do—*Freya Stark*

You have to participate relentlessly
in the manifestation of your own
blessings—*Elizabeth Gilbert*

What makes you happy?

Can you define it?

Can you communicate it?

Where do you feel the happiest? With whom? Doing what?

Visualize the scene, the sights, the sounds, the smells and tastes of what makes you happy.

Once you can define and communicate what makes you happy, make sure you're doing it as often as possible. "Relentlessly participate" in the manifestation of your happiness.

It's the little things that make
happy moments, not the grand
events. Joy comes in sips, not
gulps—*Sharon Draper*

*Reading Wayne Dyer's books and watching his programs
changed me as a person. Having him as a guest on my show
is something I will never forget.*

*One of the biggest ah-ha moments came when he asked
"How would you feel if you won the lottery?" Most people
answered that they would feel happy, free and secure. Wayne
pointed out that the feelings we expect are much easier to get
in other ways than hoping for that winning ticket.*

*What actions can you take to get the feelings a lottery win
would bring you? Look for sips of happiness, freedom, and
security each day. No purchase required.*

Once you begin to question the
truth of an inner demon, its days
are numbered—*Martha Beck*

Do you ever challenge the demons in your mind? Do you ever call bullshit on the stories you torture yourself with? Most of us don't. It would be a scary show down for sure. But vanquishing them makes you the hero of your own life. And that's a story worth telling.

One of the best ways to get real with yourself is to interact with yourself as you would a dear friend.

If your friend shared a limiting belief, a harsh self-criticism, or an outright untruth about themselves, you'd challenge them. You'd talk, cajole and maybe even be stern with them in an effort to encourage them to see the error of their thinking.

Then you'd ask them to re-frame, rethink, reexamine their faulty premise. Finally, you'd remind them to hang on to this new way of thinking.

Do that. For yourself.

Treat yourself the same way
you'd treat someone you love
and adore—*Mastin Kipp*

Let this sink in. Take it to heart. This is a game changer.

For most of us, the voice in our head is a nag, a brow beater, and a harsh critic.

These things we would not tolerate from others. Yet here we are, treating ourselves this way.

When you catch yourself, be stern and tell yourself to knock it off. Tell yourself that the person you are berating is with you through thick and thin, hardship and happiness. Remind yourself that kind of support is rare indeed.

Start a new conversation in your head. You are your own most cherished companion, to be loved and adored.

We either make ourselves
miserable or we make ourselves
strong—the amount of work is
the same—*Carlos Castenada*

A friend sent me a thought-provoking blog post by her friend, artist Dreama Perry, about poo cupcakes. That's right. Poo. Cupcakes.

Here's the premise: If I offered you a cupcake and explained that there was just a bit of poo in it—just a very little bit—would you eat it? Of course not! Even the littlest bit of something nasty can contaminate the whole of everything!

How often do you let a little fear, a little doubt, a pinch of insecurity, just a taste of worry spoil your outlook? Harm your relationships? Impinge upon your true life?

There was a study on women's attitudes toward food, involving French and American women. They were shown images and asked to say the first thing that came to mind. One of the images was a gorgeous chocolate cake. The French women all said words that meant "celebration". The American women said words that meant "Guilt" and " Bad for me"

So here's my question. Are your thoughts more like the French women? Or the American women? Are your thoughts healing? Or hurtful? You control those thoughts. Nobody else does.

Life is a constant series of choices. Whether it's saying yes when we mean no, judging ourselves or others, being overwhelmed with worry or fear, or listening to the voice in your head, choose the good thing.

Put down the poison....and don't settle for the Poo Cupcake!

Leave your front door and your
back door open. Let thoughts
come and go. Just don't serve
them tea—*Shunryu Suzuki*

Our minds become so entangled in the constant chatter, judging, and worrying about the actions of others and ourselves.

We need to learn to let the flow of thoughts come and go without getting tangled in them. Take the stance that people are inherently capable and able to manage their lives, just as we can manage our own.

There's no need to mentally weigh in on every encounter; instead, let all the thoughts breeze through. Let them pass without giving in to the urge to offer them tea.

You need to learn how to select
your thoughts just the same way you
select your clothes every day. This
is a power you can cultivate. If you
want to control things in your life
so bad, work on the mind. That's
the only thing you should be trying
to control *–Richard, Eat Pray Love*

Nobody gets buff without working out. Nobody becomes fluent without studying the language. Nobody gets fed without putting food in their cupboard.

Everything takes effort. But the effort diminishes over time, while the desired outcome becomes the state of being. Buff. Fluent. Fed.

The same goes with your mind. Sure it's hard at first to train your thoughts to be only those that serve you. But with time, you and your mind can sync up. And that's the only thing you should try to control.

Relax, and once a day, at least
Contrive to be a perfect beast!
Free, uninhibited, untamed,
Unscrupulous and unashamed.
In short, a normal man or woman
Instead of something superhuman!
—*Rolfe Humphries*

This was a favorite quote of my grandmother and my great grandmother. I love it more than I can say.

This freedom, this raw authenticity, is how we connect with our human-ness.

Honoring our primal instincts and our noble aspirations makes us full and complete. The trick is finding that balance of uninhibited existence and the pursuit of our higher selves. No one said it would be easy!

The attempt to develop a sense
of humor and to see things in a
humorous light is some kind of a
trick learned while mastering the
art of living—*Viktor E. Frankl*

The first time I read this it stopped me in my tracks. Viktor Frankl was a Holocaust survivor and author of "Man's Search for Meaning" One of the things you'll discover when you read about him is that "in reality, this represented a short period in his long life".

That statement says so much. While most of us will never witness and endure the horrors that Mr. Frankl did, he did not define his life by the tragedy.

Instead he turned his focus to the search for meaning. To suggest that humor is a trick to the art of living should pierce your mind and stay there. Life will present all kinds of tragedies, horrors, frustrations and setbacks. Master the skill of seeing things in a humorous light.

Be aware that the problems that most of us experience are minor in the grand scheme and simply part of the human experience.

If you want to test your memory,
try to recall what you were
worrying about one year ago
today—*E. Joseph Cossman*

Your track record for getting through tough stuff is 100%. The world has yet to swallow you up. Worrying does nothing to change outcomes. It just eats away at our peace of mind. Acknowledge your worries. Write them down, Talk about them with someone you trust. Meditate to increase your equanimity muscle. Then let them go. Free yourself of the weight of worry. What have you got to lose?

Then I walked away, and I did not look back.
I had written my troubles on the sand. The
tide was coming in—*Arthur Gordon Webster*

You are comprised of 84 minerals, 23
Elements, and 8 gallons of water Spread
across 38 trillion cells. You have been built
up from nothing by the spare parts of the
Earth you have consumed, according to
a set of instructions hidden in a double
helix and small enough to be carried by a
sperm. You are recycled butterflies, plants,
rocks, streams, firewood, wolf fur, and
shark teeth, broken down to their smallest
parts and rebuilt into our planet's most
complex living thing. You are not living
on Earth. You are Earth—*Aubrey Marcus*

*When I walk in the woods, I feel so alive and peaceful. I feel
at home. I have the same feeling walking along a coastline. It
makes sense, doesn't it? Each of us has sprung from the earth
itself, we're made of the same stuff and each of us will, when
we die, contribute to future life that the earth puts forth.*

*Finding consistent moments of "homecoming" in nature leads
to increased happiness and lower levels of anxiety, depression
and stress. It helps us to be more creative and calmer, too.
When people spend time in nature, they tend to take better
care of both themselves and their earth.*

*Go ahead, get out there and hug a tree. It'll do you both a
world of good.*

Our thoughts shape us; we become what we think. When the mind is pure, joy follows like a shadow that never leaves—*Buddha*

Tell everyone you know "My happiness depends on me, so you're off the hook."—*Esther Abraham-Hicks*

Inspired by Wayne Dyer, I started to think about a single word that would capture how I wanted my life to feel. I spent time reflecting, playing out different "what if" scenarios to find a word that truly resonated with me.

The word I chose was joy.

I realized that if my family was healthy and happy, I would feel joy. If I was healthy and fulfilled, I would feel joy. If my friendships, career, and community interactions were harmonious, I would feel joy. If the world was at peace, I'd feel joy. This one word embraced everything that mattered to me.

To keep myself focused on joy, I ask myself, "Is what I'm doing right now bringing me joy? If not, then why the hell am I doing it?"

I use small reminders to reconnect with this touchstone. Whenever I see repeating numbers on the clock—1:11, 2:22, 3:33, and so on—I pause and remember my goal is joy. When I encounter something petty or frustrating, I stop and ask: Will indulging in this bring me joy?

Choosing a word to guide you is a powerful practice. My family and I choose a new word each year, and it has become a tradition that centers us, keeps us focused, and moves us toward our personal versions of joy. What's your word?

Success isn't about how your life
looks to others. It's about how it
feels to you—*Michelle Obama*

Too many people spend money
they haven't earned, to buy things
they don't want, to impress people
they don't like—*Will Rogers*

Everyone wants to be admired and respected by others. Sometimes we need to examine our motives. There's a fine line between seeking admiration and respect vs. seeking envy and jealousy. One is admirable and respectable. The other is not.

We should actually put the responsibility for that admiration and respect on ourselves.

The best way to do that is to do what you are called to do, to be who you are called to be and to work on your own character. That's where the good stuff happens.

Change the way you look at
things and the things you look
at change—*Wayne Dyer*

What you focus on expands, and when
you focus on the goodness in your life,
you create more of it. Opportunities,
relationships, even money flowed my way
when I learned to be grateful no matter
what happened in my life—*Oprah Winfrey*

Have you ever been driving and thought there are more than the usual number of red cars on the road? And suddenly it seems all you see are red cars? The really funny thing is that your passenger may be thinking the same thing about blue ones.

You see what you want to see. You hear what you want to hear. You believe what you want to believe. If you want to see the good in your life, start by focusing on it. It's that simple.

When you make a conscious decision to pay attention and be grateful for the positives, even the most insignificant ones, you'll notice more and more show up in your life. Your mind will begin to seek out the positives without needing to be directed.

We're like magnets, we attract what we focus on—and by focusing on the good, you'll bring more of it into your life.

Carry out a random act of kindness, with no expectation of reward, safe in the knowledge that one day someone might do the same for you—*Princess Diana*

Kindness is more important than wisdom, and the recognition of this is the beginning of wisdom—*Theodore Isaac Rubin*

A single act of kindness throws out roots in all directions, and the roots spring up and make new trees—*Amelia Earhart*

Three things in human life are important. The first is to be kind. The second is to be kind. And the third is to be kind—*Henry James*

Because that's what kindness is. It's not doing something for someone else because they can't, but because you can—*Andrew Iskander*

Throw kindness around like confetti—*Unknown*

I'm kind of embarrassed to share this little tidbit: I set a calendar reminder that says, "do something nice for someone" I like to think I am a kind person, even without the reminder. But the reminder is because, like it or not, the world is filled with kind people who forget to be kind.

We're busy, distracted and focused on ourselves. My calendar reminder is just the nudge I need to send a text, make a call, mail a card, give a gift, give a hug or lend a hand. So, consider this your reminder. Do something nice for someone.

A great attitude becomes a great
mood, which becomes a great day,
which becomes a great year, which
becomes a great life—*Zig Ziglar*

The greatest discovery of all
time is that a person can change
their future by merely changing
their attitude—*Oprah Winfrey*

Our attitudes have a powerful impact on our health, well-being, stress levels, the quality of our relationships, workplace culture and the level of success we reach there.

A positive attitude shapes our perception of the world around us.

How to maintain a positive attitude? Just start.

Start being grateful. Start moving negative people out of your inner circle. Start moving positive people in. Start moving your body. Start stretching your mind. Start positive self-talk. Start all these things and then never stop.

A great life depends on it.

Let go of something today that you
no longer need—something that
is draining your energy without
providing benefit to you or anyone
you love—*Arianna Huffington*

Maybe it's self-talk. Maybe it's clutter. Whatever it is, it's weighing you down.

Working through and getting rid of the things you don't need will free up new space. Guard that space carefully. No need to refill it completely.

Space, be it mental or physical, is liberating. Keep as much as you can.

Let us decide on the route that we
wish to take to pass our life, and
attempt to sow that route with
flowers—*Madame du Chatelet*

My parents told us, "leave every place better than you found it". If our own route is more beautiful, others will be, too.

Embrace the idea that our actions can create a ripple effect of positivity.

A kind word, a courteous gesture, a donation, or a repair, each has the power to turn our world into a sprawling expanse of blooms.

Shouldn't we at least try?

I went to a monastery in Thailand.
We took our baths in the stream, we
begged for our food in the streets,
I shaved my head and walked
barefoot. My head monk asked how
it was walking. I said it hurt without
shoes. And he said, "It hurts on the
foot that's down, but the one that's
up feels really good—so focus on
that one." And I realized that all
pain and pleasure is where you put
your attention—*Deepak Chopra:*

Wow. Imagine if we did that in every aspect of our lives—relationships, work, how we see ourselves—things would change for the better.

But the difference between knowing and doing is huge. The urge to dwell on the negative looms large. Why not start small?

Set aside a bit of time each day, like during family dinners or your daily commute, to consciously notice the good stuff. It's everywhere.

Making small shifts in focus can lead to some profound life changes.

Each day is a small lifetime. Live
a good life today—*James Clear*

The only moment you are guaranteed is this one right now.

Keeping that truth firmly in the forefront of our minds isn't fatal thinking. It's how we remain grateful and mindful by making the most of the only day we know we have.

Tell your family and friends that you love them. Really savor your morning coffee. Eat delicious food. Find something wonderful to read, watch, listen to. Walk in the woods. Ditch the doom scrolling. Get out of your comfort zone. Get off autopilot.

Live a good life today. And tomorrow? Repeat.

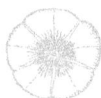

It's a funny thing about life, once
you begin to take note of the
things you are grateful for, you
begin to lose sight of the things
that you lack—*Germany Kent*

Have you ever taken a gratitude walk? It involves acknowledging something you're thankful for with each step.

I gave it a try and was amazed at the endless list beyond the obvious like health and family.

From sunglasses to toothpaste, remote controls to elevators, and even a light breeze—appreciating these everyday comforts can be truly eye-opening.

Give it a go and witness how it shifts your perspective, even if just for a moment.

Silent gratitude isn't much use
to anyone—*Gertrude Stein*

Think about a favorite childhood memory and all the people involved in it.

Think about a teacher or coach that really impacted you.

Think about a friend who was there for you when you needed them most. A neighbor that's always there to lend a hand—or a cup of sugar. Think about your family. Your colleagues. The lady who does the repairs at the dry cleaner.

Most of us have a whole lot of gratitude and appreciation for the people in our lives. But do those people know how we feel?

Close your eyes and imagine how good they'd feel if they knew. Now make it real: Tell them.

We often take for granted the
very things that most deserve
our gratitude—*Cynthia Ozick*

How often do you actually count your blessings?

You are breathing. You have people who love you. You are well fed. You have a home. Those of us who can say any of these four blessings that are so lucky.

If you take a mental inventory of all the people and things you encounter or utilize each day without a second thought, it's an embarrassment of riches.

Give it all some gratitude and notice how good that feels. There's science behind that good feeling. Gratitude boosts your mood, supports better health and increases happiness. And that deserves some more gratitude—which in turn produces more gratitude.

This is one cycle you don't want to break. Keep this good thing going.

If the only prayer you ever
say is thank you, that will be
enough—*Meister Eckhart*

Think about how life supports you every day. How much is available to you without even having to ask. Being aware of just how much we are supported can open the door to more abundance and release in you a sense of gratitude and generosity.

How many times have you gotten just what you need, just when you needed it, with no effort on your part? How many times have you been on the receiving end of unexpected support or kindness? Consciously remember these times. Keep them in rotation on your emotional playlist. Expect them to continue. Look for them. Be grateful for them.

Think about the people who have helped you in the everyday moments, and when you needed it most. Think about the many things you've been given.

Equally important is to think about the times you were the one helping and giving. That should be on repeat in your mind, too. Continue the flow of receiving—and giving and be grateful for both.

Committing to a daily gratitude practice can take your life to places you never dreamed about. I promise you'll be grateful you did.

I grow little of the food I eat, and of the little I
do grow I did not breed or perfect the seeds.

I do not make any of my own clothing.

I speak a language I did not invent or refine.

I did not discover the mathematics I use.

I am protected by freedoms and laws
I did not conceive of or legislate, and
do not enforce or adjudicate.

I am moved by music I did not create myself.

When I needed medical attention, I
was helpless to help myself survive.

I did not invent the transistor, the
microprocessor, object oriented programming,
or most of the technology I work with.

I love and admire my species, living and dead,
and am totally dependent on them for my life
and well-being—*Steve Jobs, in an email to himself*

Appreciation can make a day, even
change a life—*Margaret Cousins*

*As individuals, as families, as communities, and as countries,
it's easy to be our own little island. But we are not.*

*Echoing Steve Jobs observation, take a look around wherever
you are right now.*

*How much of what you see are you responsible for inventing,
creating, building, growing, harvesting, packaging, shipping?
What would you do without these things?*

*How much respect and gratitude do you consciously feel for the
many unseen, unsung people from all around the world that
add to the creature comforts you enjoy on your "little island"?*

We need each other. Let's remind ourselves to act accordingly.

A well-spent day brings happy
sleep—*Leonardo DaVinci*

When training hospitality and event teams, I make the point that what we're truly selling is more than a service; it's how guests "feel when they walk out the door".

I want them to reflect on their experience as they head to their car, thinking about how good it was.

This quote, and indeed this book, shares that same message: live each day with the intention of getting into bed at night and reflecting on how good it was.

Then, wake up the next morning and do it again.

A single event can awaken within
us a stranger totally unknown
to us. To live is to be slowly
born—*Antoine de Saint-Exupéry*

As I write this, I'm awaiting the birth of my very first grandbaby. I'm so moved by my child having a child.

The birth of my own children changed me so profoundly that I can only imagine the countless ways this new "stranger" will awaken emotions and insights within me as a grandmother.

I'm awestruck by the potential in front of the sweet little rosebud making her debut into the world.

I'm moved by the sense of all our love and prayers and hope focused on this sweet new life and her adoring mommy and daddy.

My granddaughter is not the only one being born today. All of us who love her already are being slowly reborn, too.

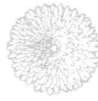

It has long been an axiom of mine
that the little things are infinitely the
most important—*Arthur Conan Doyle*

The idea that there is some "big thing" that is the key to our happiness and contentment is simply not true.

In reality, the foundation of a satisfying life is built from the seemingly small, everyday moments that we often overlook.

A good meal with friends, belly laughs, deep and meaningful relationships, a walk in nature and the feeling of a job well done—these are the quiet experiences that create a joyful life.

Become conscious of these occurrences in your daily life—they are the very essence of what makes it rich and meaningful.

It's true; the little things are actually very big indeed.

Savor your morning coffee; Take a moment and really enjoy it. Smell it. Taste it. Appreciate it. Research shows savoring—appreciating the good moments—is what separates the happiest people from the average Joe. It doesn't have to be coffee. It can be anything you do every morning. But embedding savoring in our little daily rituals is powerful. Studies show rituals matter—*Sonja Lyubomirsky*

My morning ritual is my joy: coffee, puzzles, reading, meditation, and a workout. It's my slow re-entry into the world, starting with meditation to clear my mind, followed by uplifting reading and plenty of caffeine.

The workout charges me up; reviewing my schedule frees my mind from worrying I'm missing something. This routine is non-negotiable and I honestly cherish it.

Build a morning routine that centers you, uplifts you and prepares you for the day. Embed little daily rituals and witness the power they bring.

The art of living is based on rhythm—
on give & take, ebb & flow, light &
dark, life & death. By acceptance
of all aspects of life, good & bad,
right & wrong, yours & mine, the
static, defensive life, which is what
most people are cursed with, is
converted into a dance, 'the dance of
life,' metamorphosis—*Henry Miller*

I love the line from the movie "Parenthood" when Grandma is talking about going to an amusement park and says, "I always wanted to go again. You know, it was just so interesting to me that a ride could make me so frightened, so scared, so sick, so excited, and so thrilled all together! Some didn't like it. They went on the merry-go-round. That just goes around. Nothing. I like the roller coaster. You get more out of it"

If you can really embrace this thought process, which is by no means easy to do, the dance and rhythm that both Henry Miller and Grandma describe really can be seen as a thing of heart-wrenching beauty. Even the terrifying and breathtaking parts.

To live will be an awfully big
adventure—*JM Barrie*

If there is a universal aspiration of humankind, it's to be able to look back over our lives and be satisfied with what we see.

Accomplishments, relationships and possessions are part of the big picture, of course, but I think one of the truest measuring sticks is experience and adventure.

For some folks, that may be traveling the world. For others, extreme sports. And for some people, simply exploring new sights and sounds much closer to their own community and comfort level.

Whatever and however you do it, stretch yourself in the direction of excitement and adventure. Your future self will thank you for it.

We need time to defuse, to
contemplate. Just as in sleep our
brains relax and give us dreams,
so at some time in the day we
need to disconnect, reconnect, and
look around us—*Laurie Colwin*

We tend to save this concept for vacations, weekends, and holidays.

A better strategy is to build it into your daily life. We've all heard variations on the idea that we should create lives we don't need to escape from. I embrace this whole heartedly.

Brendon Burchard takes a break after every 50 minutes of work. Oprah keeps Sundays for herself. You can do something as simple as walk a nearby park, a forest, or a shoreline.

John Burroughs said "I go to nature to be soothed, healed and have my senses put in order." Amen.

There are so many ways to bring the mindset of disconnect/ reconnect into your daily life. Find some that work for you and make them non-negotiable.

Almost everything will work again
if you unplug it for a few minutes,
including you—*Anne Lamott*

Sometimes the most productive thing
you can do is relax—*Mark Black*

The mind should be allowed some
relaxation, that it may return to its
work all the better for the rest—*Seneca*

My calendar overflows with meetings, tasks, and commitments, and I try hard not to break them. After all, I've made a commitment and that matters to me.

I also fill my calendar with ample downtime for myself, with plenty of space to do the things I love. Yet I'll swap those out with other commitments so fast it makes my head spin.

Going forward, I'm making a conscious effort (and I urge you to do the same), to value my downtime as much as my work and commitments.

It matters. Downtime makes your work time better, and vice versa.

I always encourage my kids to design their ideal life. Would anyone design their dream life without including ample time to rest, relax, and play? Certainly not. And neither should you.

CHAPTER SIX

Choosing Optimism

*Finding Hope in
Everyday Moments*

When you devote time and energy
to noticing, new doors open.
Serendipity accelerates. You feel
like the universe is conspiring to
support you. But really, you're just
not limiting yourself—*Katia Verresen*

I read a story about a woman who noted that she and her husband were in the not-so-uncommon habit of spending their evenings telling each other about all the bad things that happened during their day.

So they made a pact to flip the script and only share the good things. Soon they started to purposefully look for good things to share.

You've probably already guessed the outcome. They were amazed at how the good things started piling up. Notice the good things. Talk about them.

Open the door to limitless possibilities.

Each one leads to more

We can choose to commit to a
recursive and infinite path that
elegantly creates more of the same.

We can choose possibility.

We can choose connection.

We can choose optimism.

We can choose justice.

We can choose kindness.

We can choose resilience.

And we can decide to take responsibility.

Each leads to more of the same.

—Seth Godin

This makes me think of the alphabet game on car trips. When you're searching for a Q, you will eventually find one. It's your only focus. Other letters become less important.

If you focus your life experience on possibility, optimism and resilience, you'll find them, too.

Decide where you're going to look and stay focused.

Most of us are just about as
happy as we make up our minds
to be.—*Abraham Lincoln*

Be optimistic. Be positive. Be happy.

Start each day believing that it will be a good one, then do your part to make it so. Try to make it so. Act to make it so.

This will create a loop of optimism that will make you feel better, look better, succeed better and relate to others better than if you don't make this choice.

You are responsible for your happiness. It comes from within. Having said that, you make choices about the things you allow into your life that will impact your happiness.

Good, strong relationships add to your happiness. Healthy habits add to your happiness. Positive experiences add to your happiness. Another person, or possession, cannot make you happy in and of themselves.

Your happiness begins and ends with you.

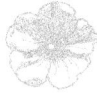

Beyond each impenetrable expanse
of thundercloud obscurity reigns
a boundless canopy of brilliant
sapphire blue—*Cara Fox*

*It's so cool to literally experience this when flying. To ascend
through rainy, cloudy skies, then break through into a beautiful
blue expanse.*

*As an analogy for life, this is spot on. There is light and dark in
everything. Neither lasts forever.*

Some of you say, "Joy is greater than sorrow," and others say, "Nay, sorrow is the greater." But I say unto you, they are inseparable. Together they come, and when one sits alone with you at your board, remember that the other is asleep upon your bed."—*Kahlil Gibran, The Prophet*

If I could define enlightenment briefly I would say it is the quiet acceptance of what is—*Wayne Dyer*

The wisdom and confidence to accept this reality, with both its optimism and pessimism sitting comfortably side by side, is a milestone in personal development.

You'll be building your inner peace.

The basis of optimism is sheer terror
—*Oscar Wilde*

Optimism is usually defined as a belief that
things will go well. But that's incomplete.
Sensible optimism is a belief that the odds are
in your favor, and over time things will balance
out to a good outcome even if what happens in
between is filled with misery. And in fact you
know it will be filled with misery. You can be
optimistic that the long-term growth trajectory
is up and to the right, but equally sure that
the road between now and then is filled with
landmines, and always will be. Those two things
are not mutually exclusive—*Morgan Housel*

I am so far from being a pessimist…on
the contrary, in spite of my scars, I am
tickled to death at life—*Eugene O'Neill*

When I read these quotes, I feel like I've found my kindred spirits.

I believe that the odds are in my favor, yet I know I will experience
misery.

This vantage point allows me to get from peak to peak…even
though I know I'll traverse dark valleys.

Don't waste your energy by being surprised by this. Accept this
reality and embrace that you couldn't possibly enjoy the view
from the mountain tops nearly so much if you hadn't endured
the cold chill of the lows. It'll make the journey so much easier—
maybe even exciting.

We are all in the gutter, but some of us
are looking at the stars—*Oscar Wilde*

It's a universal truth that each and every human walks this earth with their share of struggles, hardships, fears and insecurities. Every single one. There is no exception.

It's also true that some people, despite these things, decide to remain positive and focused on the beauty, joy and possibility that exists alongside their challenges.

Be one of them. Look up. The sky is full of stars.

Hope can be a powerful force. Maybe there's no actual magic in it, but when you know what you hope for most and hold it like a light within you, you can make things happen, almost like magic—*Laini Taylor*

There have been times in my life when I truly felt that magic is real—when things just seem to fall into place. Doors open, unexpected opportunities arise, new friendships blossom and moments of beauty and laughter appear around every corner.

Interestingly, these magical periods always align with times when my mind and heart are open. When I am actively expecting, willing, and dreaming these things into existence.

That's the key: holding hope "like a light within you," tending to it, and cultivating it. When you maintain this mindset, it has a remarkable way of turning dreams into reality.

*You **can** make things happen.*

It is madness to hate all roses because
you got scratched with one thorn. To
give up on your dreams because one
didn't come true. To lose faith in prayers
because one was not answered, to give up
on our efforts because one of them failed.
It's foolish to condemn friends because
one betrayed you. To not believe in love
because someone was unfaithful and to
throw away chances to be happy because
you didn't succeed on the first try. There
will always be another opportunity,
another friend, another love, a new
force. For every end, there is always a
new beginning—*Antoine de Saint-Exupéry*

This passage from "The Little Prince" is packed full of truth and hope and wisdom.

Keep the faith. Just keep it. There is so much that occurs in a full life.

All of our experiences are useful. Everything shapes us. Let it.

A dream is the bearer of a new possibility, the enlarged horizon, the great hope—*Howard Thurman*

I wanted a lemon tree for many years. I bought one once. It was a little twig, shorter than my forearm, with a smattering of leaves. It didn't amount to much, and I lost interest in it. After a couple of months I dumped it in the compost pile. But that didn't stop my dream of a lemon tree.

I was out with a friend recently and we stopped into a plant shop. I asked about lemon trees. I explained my desire for a larger tree, not a little stick, and that I dreamt of harvesting my own lemons.

Here's the thing. I can picture this. I can see it as if it's real life. I really want this to happen.

The woman who owned the shop said she'd keep her eye out for a lemon tree for me and sure enough, a few weeks later she called to say she had one in the shop. I became the hopeful, excited owner of a 5-foot-tall lemon tree.

This time around my dream is clearer, my resolve for it coming true more focused. That in turn has moved me to research how to care for my tree. How to water, fertilize and light it.

Each morning after I finish my writing, the first thing I do is go check on my tree.

Guess what? It's blooming right and left! And now I know how to pollinate those blooms when they're ready. I am brimming with hope and possibility.

Not all my dreams are about lemon trees. But the ones that have traction include envisioning them, really seeing them happen, maintaining a focus on them and nurturing them with love and attention.

Will I harvest armloads of lemons from my tree? We'll see. But I'm following this dream with great gusto. And I hope you follow yours that way too.

Ah, but a man's reach should exceed his grasp, Or what's a heaven for?—*Robert Browning*

The only thing standing between you and your goal is the bullshit story you keep telling yourself as to why you can't achieve it—*Jordan Belfort*

I read an insightful article about our tendency to not get our hopes up—just in case. As in, "I don't want to get my hopes up".

Why do we do this? What does it do for us? Not one thing.

Yes, getting our hopes up is risky. What we want may not happen. But why not spend your thoughts on excitement and hope rather than despair and defeat?

You will or you won't have your hopes dashed. Preemptive doubt only robs us of the excitement of anticipation.

Go on, get your hopes up. Reach beyond your grasp. What if it all works out? It could just be heaven.

When I despair, I remember that all
through history the way of truth and
love have always won. There have
been tyrants and murderers, and for
a time, they can seem invincible, but
in the end, they always fall. Think
of it—always—*Mahatma Gandhi*

One of my favorite lines from a Marianne Williamson prayer is "I do not stop my eyes at the veil of horror that surrounds the world, but rather I extend my vision to the possibilities for love for myself and others."

There is so much horror, violence, anger, inequity, fear and hatred in this world. We can't stop our eyes from it.

But we can consider, and have faith, that in the end truth and love can win.

Behind me is infinite power, before
me is endless possibility, around me is
boundless opportunity—*Mac Anderson*

If we could embrace this mindset all the time, imagine the positive changes it could bring to our lives! It would change your outlook. Your approach. Your choices. Your mood.

But what holds us back? It's that nagging voice of fear in our heads.

When you're choosing your life support system, ditch that negative voice and surround yourself with infinite power, endless possibility and boundless opportunity instead.

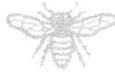

Open yourself wide to
all the universe has to
say—*Melody Beattie*

Each quote I've gathered over the last decade leads to a cascade of related ones, which drives home the point of repeated wisdom offered through the ages.

There is a force, a power, an awesome energy that is available to each of us. Don't disregard it. Don't take it for granted. Open your eyes, your ears, your heart. It's everywhere. And it's yours.

There are only two ways to
live your life. One is as though
nothing is a miracle. The
other is as though everything
is a miracle—*Albert Einstein*

The sun rises and sets without fail. The tides come in and out. Babies. Galaxies. Flowers.

It's near impossible to get through a day without seeing something miraculous—not to mention all the things we don't see. It's easy to saunter past miracle upon miracle every day without a second glance.

Remind yourself that everything is a miracle, including you.

Sometimes your only available
transportation is a leap of
faith—*Margaret Shepard*

Surrender your worry, fear and
doubt to your creator. Allow a
miracle to show up in a most
unexpected way—*Unknown*

*What stops you from taking a leap of faith? What prevents you
from surrendering your worry, fear and doubt? Why can't a
miracle show up for you?*

*These are not rhetorical questions. These are things you
absolutely should question.*

*What has worry, fear or doubt done for you anyway? What if
you dropped them and chose instead to just breathe and use
faith as your preferred mode of transport?*

Turn negativity into positive action. Take one thing today that you feel negative about. Before the day is out, take one positive action that diminishes the negativity. Such actions include the following: standing up for yourself, speaking your truth, fixing what can be fixed, asking for help, seeking wise advice, walking away from things that can't be fixed, reducing the stress and looking at your role in creating the negative situation. But the possibilities are endless. Taking even a small action begins to change the feedback you're getting—*Deepak Chopra*

When your day has gone astray, remind yourself that it doesn't mean your life has done so, too.

Nobody gets a pass from the occasional bad day.

It's your response that can turn the day around or allow it to fester.

It's completely up to you. How would you like to feel?

The choice is yours.

CHAPTER SEVEN

Unshakeable Strength

Building Resilience Through Life's Challenges

When the storm rips you to pieces,
you get to decide how to put yourself
back together again—*Bryant McGill*

All the adversity I've had in my life, all my
troubles and obstacles, have strengthened
me...You may not realize it when it happens,
but a kick in the teeth may be the best
thing in the world for you—*Walt Disney*

I spoke once on a panel of women discussing second acts. I anchored my comments around the word Lifequakes, a term coined by Bruce Fieler. I had Bruce as a guest on my show years ago to chat about his book "The Council of Dads". While that isn't the book that birthed the phrase Lifequake, the experience described in it was a lifequake of major proportion. I encourage you to check it out. Spoiler alert—you will cry.

Lifequakes as a topic for our panel grew out of a pre-event discussion with our moderator, who offered her condolences on the loss of my husband. I mentioned to her how stunned I was to discover that the average age a woman becomes a widow in the US is 58 years old. That's how old I was when my husband died. That was a lifequake.

But recognizing that everyone has lifequakes, and that my young widowhood was not unusual, helped me keep things in perspective. It's all part of the human condition.

Life quakes can be:
   Losing a spouse
   Having a child
   Ending a relationship
   Getting married
   Getting a medical diagnosis
   Undertaking a move

We all experienced a collective lifequake during the pandemic. Covid got us all thinking about our work, our homes, our relationships and more. I don't think there's a person alive that wasn't changed by the pandemic.

Statistically, each of us goes through dozens of life quakes in our lifetime. I like to think some of them might be called "life tremors." One in 10 of these events are massive enough to be called a life quake, however, and they tend to happen about every 5 years. They're roughly 50/50 involuntary vs self induced. About half happen to you. The other half happen by choice. Almost all life quakes can find you in a better place if you approach it right.

I sometimes feel like I'm the queen of life quakes. I've launched multiple brands and businesses, created a radio show, a television show, published a cookbook and built my own consulting business. Those are all positive quakes, but quakes nonetheless. I've also had a business fail—spectacularly and publicly. But that quake, and it was a doozy, led to some of my greatest successes.

What if I told you that you can expect life quakes throughout your life? That you can work to get better at them, to handle each one more skillfully than the last? You can. You will. Especially if you try the strategies that I've used when a life quake hits:

Swim to shore—I used to say this to my daughter when she was younger. Think about a life quake as being plopped into the middle of a lake. Don't thrash. Don't panic. Swim to shore. Slow and steady. Get to a place where you can catch your breath, dry off, collect yourself. This is key. Give yourself time to take stock of what is happening.

Those things you don't want to feel? Feel them. Give yourself the time and space to feel into every corner of what you're going through. Why are you scared? Don't avoid it—go all the way in. List everything that worries you about your circumstances and allow yourself to acknowledge every bit of it. I quite literally make myself imagine every worst case scenario that could happen. Funny thing about really looking at what scares you... you realize how unlikely most of your scary scenarios are—and you realize you can handle those that might actually happen. Don't skip this step—be thorough. It's the foundation for the positive change that you need.

Free yourself from conditioning. As you reshape and define your future, pay attention to how guided you are by past conditioning. What is really true for you? What do you want? Not what your Instagram page wants. Not what your friends want. Not what your parents or children want. What do you want? Ask yourself, "Am I thinking expansively, or am I limiting myself?" and "How can I reshape my perspectives to see limitless possibilities instead of restrictions?" Think outside the box—think like there is no box—and rebuild with your ideal life in mind.

Let go of your past and step into your future. Anytime a major change happens in life, you must let go of your old identity— and that can feel very chaotic. As your vision becomes clear and you start to see progress it becomes easier to settle into the new version of yourself. And guess what? Another life quake is on its way to you. But this time, you'll recognize it's simply part of a full life. Your track record for getting through things so far is 100%. And now you've got a strategy to handle it, come what may.

The great law of nature is that it
never stops. There is no end.

When you overcome one obstacle, another
one waits in the shadows. Life is a process
of overcoming obstacles, one after the
other. The obstacle becomes the way so
you might as well enjoy it—*Ryan Holiday*

You can't live off one meal, one day of exercise, one day at work. Relationships aren't made in one encounter. Dreams aren't met with just one wish.

Every single day is a chance to begin again, with all the obstacles, setbacks and challenges of a well-lived life.

Your to-do list will never be completed. Your family will never stop having needs. Your laundry will never remain done. Your employer will never expect less than your A game.

Fighting against this reality is a losing game. Try to step into the flow of life and find music in its repetitive rhythms.

When something goes wrong in
your life, just yell "Plot twist!"
and move on—*Molly Weis*

It's easy to overestimate the significance of a single decision, outcome, or event as it's happening.

Remind yourself to take a deep breath and let it go when things don't go your way.

In the long run, your life experiences—good or bad—are the result of many small decisions, outcomes, and events stacked up over time.

We all have failures. We all have successes. The greater truth is that no single success or failure ever defines us.

When everything is charged with fear, a spark can ignite a panic. It can ensure demoralization and then defeat. But just as easily, one person can ground this dangerous electrical current. One person can turn things around.

The question for you, then, is are you that person? Are you part of the problem or can you be the solution? Are you the one they call? Or are you the one they have to calm down?—*Ryan Holiday*

The ultimate measure of your wisdom and strength is how calm you are when facing any given situation. Calmness is indeed a superpower. The ability to not overreact or take things personally keeps your mind clear and your heart at peace, which instantly gives you the upper hand—*Marc & Angel Chernoff*

In May 2022, Darren Harrison found himself in an extraordinary situation: the pilot of the plane he was a passenger on suddenly became unresponsive. With no piloting experience, Darren managed to land the plane safely.

How did he do it? Remarkably, Darren was able to keep his composure throughout the ordeal, as did the air traffic controller who guided him to the ground. Staying calm was a conscious choice for both men.

This story struck a chord with me because I'm not sure I could have remained calm in such a high-stress situation.

What stayed with me was the lesson on the power of composure in the face of panic, danger, chaos, and uncertainty.

People are sensitive to the energy around them. We all carry energy—it can be frantic, frenetic, and anxious, or solid, calm, and centered. The energy you bring to a situation can make an enormous difference—sometimes even a life-or-death difference—whether you're parenting, at work, or in everyday interactions. The tone of your voice and the words you choose are equally important.

So, when faced with a challenge that tests your ability to stay calm, remember Darren Harrison. Choose to remain calm and carry on. Your life just might depend on it.

Feeling sorry for yourself, and your
present condition, is not only a waste
of energy but the worst habit you
could possibly have—*Dale Carnegie*

Don't feel sorry for yourself. Only
assholes do that—*Haruki Murakami*

Even the most self-aware among us occasionally slip into moments of self-pity.

But that's the key—moments. They don't wallow there. They don't mope about looking for all the reasons that the world is against them.

Acknowledging your feelings and refocusing them in a more productive direction will remind you of all the reasons to be grateful instead of pitiful. You will think about how to do things differently next time.

When all else fails, they remember Murakami's advice and make the conscious choice not to be one of those people.

I dream of never being called resilient
again in my life. I'm exhausted by strength.
I want support. I want softness. I want
ease. I want to be amongst kin. Not patted
on the back for how well I take a hit. Or
for how many—*Zandashe L'Orelia Brown*

*Like most human beings, I have overcome many obstacles,
gotten over hurdles, endured heartbreak and disappointment,
even betrayal. And, like most human beings, I have come out
the other side even stronger.*

*For much of my life I loved quoting "Throw me to the wolves
and I will return leading the pack." And I usually did.*

*But now, this quote suits me better. I think it's a natural
progression of life and how we move through it. Support,
softness, ease. How lovely.*

We have to be willing to look at death, letting go,
heartbreak and chaos with the eyes of celebration,
for all these things are a part of the dance of creation
that keeps Life moving. There is something to
be found in what we have lost—*Mastin Kipp*

The only way to make sense of change
is to plunge into it, move with it,
and join the dance—*Alan Watts*

Life isn't about waiting for the storm to pass…It's
about learning to dance in the rain—*Vivian Greene*

My husband was injured in surgery and, after many months, died as a result. It was an excruciating time for all of us. The pain, the uncertainty, the exhaustion, the worry—our family was plunged into an extended hell that I wish upon no one. During this time, the kids would ask me questions I couldn't answer. We all had emotions we had not had before. We were navigating unknown waters. It was terrifying.

I happened to hear Brene Brown talk about FFTs (effing first times) and it was like a gift. Having this simple phrase as a touchstone helped us all tremendously. It allowed us to be vulnerable and honest. None of us, our children or their parents, had been through this before. It was an FFT for all of us. Our experience also uncovered in each of us a new level of strength and courage. It showed me just what we were all made of. There were glimmers of beauty peeking through the horror.

That's the thing about life—it's the effing first time for each and every one of us. Knowing that life can be both brutal and beautiful, I hope, nonetheless, you dance.

Life is not always a matter of holding
good cards, but sometimes, playing
a poor hand well—*Jack London*

We cannot change the cards we are dealt,
just how we play the hand—Randy Pausch

Play the hand you're dealt like it's the one
you've aways wanted—*Inky Johnson*

One of the things I love about quotes is the recurring themes within them. Each author's spin gives me fuller context. When the core message is the same, that tells me it's solid wisdom.

No one—not one single human that has ever walked the earth—is exempt from misfortune, or the occasional bad hand. The people who inspire us, who leave a mark, play through knowing that they can either endure it or make it work to their advantage. When life deals you one of these, and it will, keep in mind that your next hand may well be a royal flush.

You've got to know when to hold 'em
Know when to fold 'em
Know when to walk away
And know when to run
You never count your money
When you're sittin' at the table
There'll be time enough for countin'
When the dealin's done.

The Gambler *by Kenny Rogers*

You will lose someone you can't live
without, and your heart will be badly
broken, and the bad news is that you
never completely get over the loss of your
beloved. But this is also the good news.
They live forever in your broken heart
that doesn't seal back up. And you come
through. It's like having a broken leg that
never heals perfectly—that still hurts
when the weather gets cold, but you learn
to dance with the limp—*Anne Lamot*t

*I lost my mother when I was in my twenties. I thought I would
never get over her loss. And I didn't. I told people way back
then that it was like a hole was blown right through me, but
eventually I got used to the breeze.*

*When my husband died my kids were not much older than I
was when I lost my mom. I knew what they were going through
and yet I was going through a whole new kind of loss.*

*Here's the thing about grief, it comes in many shapes and sizes.
It comes more than once. No one can escape it. But somehow,
we all survive it.*

In life you will meet two kinds of people.
Ones who build you up, and ones who
tear you down. But in the end, you
will thank them both—*Unknown*

I truly believe that those folks who tear you down actually build you up more in the long run.

I have learned the most searingly valuable lessons by realizing who and what I don't want to be from those who have torn me down. I've used the examples set by the same people as a measuring stick against which I make sure I never measure.

I've learned objectivity, compassion and kindness from some of the most jaded, mean-spirited people I've encountered. And here's the funny thing: over the years there are fewer and fewer of them in my path.

Those same people that tore me down taught me the value of boundaries and an intolerance for allowing them any space in my life.

Next time someone tears you down, mentally thank them and walk away, taking only the lesson in how not to be along with you.

Tragedy should be used as a source
of strength—*Tibetan philosophy*

I saw something on Instagram recently about how all strong people have gone through very difficult times.

I know it's true. I lost my mother in my early 20's, I became a widow in my late 50's. I lost a business. I lost a job.

But with each challenge, another layer of strength and resiliency has been added.

I am grateful that I have learned, beyond a shadow of a doubt, that every problem, every setback, every loss comes bearing its own gift.

Embrace this truth as you experience life's guaranteed ups and downs.

The more you trust your intuition,
the more empowered you become,
the stronger you become, and the
happier you become—*Gisele Bundchen*

Trust your instincts. Intuition
doesn't lie—*Oprah Winfrey*

If prayer is you talking to God, then intuition
is God talking to you—*Wayne Dyer*

It's incredible that every human being is endowed with the quiet superpower of intuition. We all have a "sense" that tells us so much.

In my experience intuition is rarely wrong, yet we underutilize it. When we experience the sting of an unwanted outcome, we all say "I knew I shouldn't have (fill in the blank)" We knew, but we didn't trust ourselves.

Intuition is powerful. Intuition is real. Next time, trust your gut. It only wants the best for you!

If you ever find yourself in the
wrong story, leave—*Mo Willems*

I remember in my late 20s, I was riding in the car with my Dad. I was going through some tough stuff and I said, "Somehow I've ended up in the wrong life."

His response was, "That's how you build a backbone, being baptized by fire." That was so unlike anything he would usually say.

It dawned on me later that someone had likely once said the same thing to him. It didn't give me much comfort that day, but it stayed with me and I have learned how right he was.

The very best parts of me all stem from the very hardest times in my life. If you're going through hell, take comfort that it's building your backbone. It's honing your resolve and pointing you where you need to go. But don't stay there. If you're in the wrong story, leave.

CHAPTER EIGHT

The Courage to Thrive

Boldly Stepping Into Your Life

The first rule is to keep an untroubled
spirit. The second is to look things
in the face and know them for
what they are—*Marcus Aurelius*

This is a bit of a chicken-or-egg scenario. You can't have one without the other.

I've learned that avoidance of anything, be it worries, obligations or tough conversations, creates more stress and anxiety than facing it head on.

Face your demons. You can vanquish them more easily than you give yourself credit for.

There's an untroubled spirit waiting on the other side. That's a payoff worth working for.

A life lived in fear is a life half
lived—*Baz Luhrmann*

Courage is faith that has said its
prayers—*Dorothy Bernard*

My Mom died of breast cancer before my kids were born. Losing my parents was one of my worst fears, and it came true.

I was scared. I thought I would die, too. I thought my father, brothers and sisters might die.

Once I became a mother, I was terrified that I would die as my mom did and leave them motherless.

I lived in such fear of it that each year the idea of my annual mammogram paralyzed me. I went to each appointment like I was going to the electric chair, imagining my motherless babies. The fears multiplied. I kept a fear-focus for many years.

One evening we watched the Australian film "Strictly Ballroom". Baz's quote is a line from the movie. Like a lightning bolt, it changed my life. "A life lived in fear is a life half lived"

I suddenly understood. I knew I wanted a full life. Fear had done nothing for me—except make me fearful.

Now, I focus on bravery instead. Faith, courage and bravery are all wrapped up in each other.

Let fear go. No fear. Live a full life.

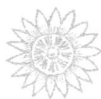

When you argue with reality, you lose—but only 100 percent of the time—*Byron Katie*

What's worrying you? How do you need to do better? What do you need to stop doing? What do you need to do more of? How are you good to yourself—and others? How are you not?

This year, vow to face things head on.

Avoidance and delusion don't get you where you want to go. And most of the things that you've avoided look much smaller in the rear view mirror.

You can do this.

Too often we duck from the tough stuff or hide in our fears. But courage is contagious—and lurks inside even the timidest. With each tough decision, the next one gets a little easier. Soon your natural impulse is to do the right thing—despite the difficulty—*Jim VandeHei*

Think about a time when you avoided something important, when you didn't step up when stepping up was the thing to do. It didn't feel good, did it?

Now recall a time when you did something challenging, uncomfortable, or impactful.. That felt pretty good.

The shirking, the ducking, the avoiding—our minds try to trick us into that being the better choice to avoid pain and discomfort.

Here's the truth—the comfort, pride and peace of mind come from courageously doing the tough stuff.

The wise man in the storm prays to
God, not for safety from danger, but
for deliverance from fear—*Emerson*

When my kids were younger, I would say the same thing each
time they'd leave the house: "Be safe, be smart, have fun"

Unfortunately, the truth is that very rarely do those three things
go together. Safe. Smart. Fun. In life, safety is not guaranteed.

The only way any of us know what fun is all about is that we've
had enough bad times to be able to tell the difference. The
only way we get smarter is to have started out a bit dumber.
Hopefully, we learn from our mistakes. But here's the kicker.
The only way we can remain completely safe is to live in a
bubble, cut off from the world. To avoid friendships, love
affairs, international travel...and shots of tequila.

You can't be in love without knowing heartbreak. You can't be
a parent without knowing fear. You can't be an entrepreneur
with knowing risk. You can't be much of anything at all
without—at some point—getting your ego bruised, your heart
broken, your knee scraped. But the alternative is even more
horrifying. No love. No risk. No fun.

Recognize that a full life is a risky proposition.

ABOUT THE AUTHOR

Amy Tobin is a "straight shooting nurturer" and dynamic leader with thirty years of experience in media, events, food, and hospitality. Passionate about creating meaningful experiences that inspire, connect, and elevate communities, she brings creativity and energy to everything she does—whether raising her family, leading a team, or designing a brand activation that leaves a lasting impact.

The former host of "Amy's Table" on Cincinnati's Q102, Amy is also the author of Amy's Table: Food for Family and Friends *and now,* Food for Thought.

www.ingramcontent.com/pod-product-compliance
Lightning Source LLC
Chambersburg PA
CBHW031429270326
41930CB00007B/629